AIDS in the

Nervous
System

AIDS in the Nervous System

Richard Lechtenberg, M.D.

Associate Professor of Clinical Neurology
Department of Neurology
State University of New York
Health Science Center at Brooklyn
College of Medicine
Chief, Division of Neurology
Long Island College Hospital
Brooklyn, New York

Joanna Hollenberg Sher, M.D.

Professor of Clinical Pathology and Distinguished Service Professor
Department of Pathology
State University of New York
Health Science Center at Brooklyn
College of Medicine
Director, Neuropathology Laboratory
Kings County Hospital Center
Brooklyn, New York

Churchill Livingstone
New York, Edinburgh, London, Melbourne   1988

Library of Congress Cataloging in Publication Data

Lechtenberg, Richard.
  AIDS in the nervous system / Richard Lechtenberg,
Joanna Hollenberg Sher.
    p. cm.
  Includes bibliographies and index.
  ISBN 0-443-08616-8
  1. Nervous system—Diseases. 2. AIDS (Disease)—
Complications and sequelae. I. Sher, Joanna
Hollenberg,   . II. Title.
  [DNLM: 1. Acquired Immunodeficiency Syndrome—
complications. 2. Nervous System Diseases—etiology.
WD 308 L459a]
RC346.L42 1988
616.97'92—dc 19
DNLM/DLC   88-14959
for Library of Congress   CIP

© **Churchill Livingstone Inc. 1988**

Distributed in the United Kingdom by Churchill
Livingstone, Robert Stevenson House, 1–3 Baxter's
Place, Leith Walk, Edinburgh EH1 3AF, and by
associated companies, branches, and representatives
throughout the world.

Accurate indications, adverse reactions, and dosage
schedules for drugs are provided in this book, but it is
possible that they may change. The reader is urged to
review the package information data of the manufacturers
of the medications mentioned.

The publishers have made every effort to trace the
copyright holders for borrowed material. If they have
inadvertently overlooked any, they will be pleased to
make the necessary arrangements at the first opportunity.

Acquisitions Editor: *Robert A. Hurley*
Copy Editor: *Kamely Dahir*
Production Designer: *Angela Cirnigliaro*
Production Supervisor: *Jocelyn Eckstein*

Printed in the United States of America

First published in 1988

To Dr. Dorothy Hollenberg
Dr. Joseph Hollenberg
and Dr. Sid Gilman

Preface

Acquired immune deficiency syndrome (AIDS) has had such a dramatic impact on the practice of medicine, it is hard to believe it first appeared fewer than ten years ago. AIDS and the virus, human immunodeficiency virus (HIV), that is responsible for AIDS cause a wide spectrum of neurologic problems. As this epidemic continues it will become increasingly important to manage those neurologic problems.

It is not just neurologists who will be called on to treat these neurologic complications. Obstetricians, neonatologists, and pediatricians are already finding their practices complicated by the newborns and children infected with HIV. The first signs of AIDS in the infant or child are often neurologic signs. Dementia may evolve rapidly in the affected child even if immunodeficiency is not evident or not substantial. Dementia and psychoses, as well as ataxia, tremors, seizures, weakness, and personality disorders are also common in adults with AIDS. Family physicians, internists, and psychiatrists are faced with an increasing number of HIV infected patients with cognitive or affective disorders from nervous system disease caused by AIDS.

This book is the combined effort of a clinician and a neuropathologist. Our objective is to help physicians to diagnosis and manage the neurologic complications of AIDS and HIV infection. We have tried to focus mainly on the neurologic diseases and disturbances that appear in individuals with AIDS, appropriate courses of management for these neurologic problems, probable complications, and usual prognosis. For those physicians who are unfamiliar with the basic mechanisms underlying and associated with AIDS, we hope the chapters on the character, epidemiology, and prevention of AIDS will provide useful perspectives.

AIDS is a rapidly evolving area of medicine; so we have based our recommendations on those courses of action where there is a consensus among the scientific community. We have tried to write a book that will be useful to all physicians who will be obliged to deal with patients suffering from the neurologic complications of AIDS.

Richard Lechtenberg, M.D.
Joanna Hollenberg Sher, M.D.

Acknowledgments

Many people contributed to this book, but those most essential to its realization were the patients at Kings County Hospital Center, Brooklyn, New York, who suffered with this tragic disease. These patients or their relatives allowed the collection of pathologic material that is reproduced in this book. The faculty and staff of the Neuropathology Laboratory at Kings County Hospital Center performed the pathologic examinations on many of the cases presented. Special thanks are due Dr. Chandrakant Rao, Dr. Archinto Anzil, and Drs. Edward Klein, Peter Kozlowski, Olga Ris, Soon-Myoung Paik, and Monica Wrzolek.

We also wish to thank our colleagues in general pathology at Kings County Hospital Center and at other Brooklyn hospitals who contributed case material to these studies. These physicians include Drs. Hosoon Dincsoy, Yvonne Lamy, Raoul Alessandri, Sundaram Sridhar, Yale Rosen, Hyun-Sook Ohm, and Nagabhushanam Nimmagadda. Ms. Antoinette Dorch did the original artwork, and Mr. Albert Paglialunga did the final photography.

Contents

Color insert appears after page 100.

The Character of AIDS

The acquired immune deficiency syndrome (AIDS) is a disturbance of the body's defenses against infection that results from an infection.[1-3] The infectious agent is a virus, and the damage it does to the immune system of most, if not all, people it infects is life-threatening.[3-5] The responsible agent has been well characterized structurally and is called the human immunodeficiency virus or HIV. It has several unusual traits, including an affinity for specific lymphocytes in the human immune system and a tendency to diversify into an extraordinary number of immunologically distinct strains.[6-8] The basis for this structural variability and the conditions necessary for the virus (HIV) to cause lethal complications remain poorly understood. Previously healthy individuals who acquire HIV become susceptible to opportunistic infections and die after months or years of recurrent infections.[9] To have AIDS, an individual must be infected with HIV and must have immune system damage secondary to or other lesions typical of that infection.[3]

Many organ systems are damaged by the recurrent infections that develop with AIDS, but damage to the central nervous system is especially common.[10-12] Systemic infections, particularly those affecting the lungs, kidneys, gastrointestinal tract, and skin, may respond to conventional antibiotic treatment; but disease developing in the central nervous system is often refractory, disabling, and fatal.[3,13] Two factors specifically increase the destructiveness of the human immunodeficiency virus in the nervous system: (1) the immune barriers usually protecting the nervous system work to its disadvantage when infections develop in the nervous system in patients with AIDS, and (2) the virus that causes AIDS attacks the nervous system directly, in addition to attacking the immune system.[14-16]

The initial experience with AIDS in the United States suggested that a relatively limited segment of the population would be affected by this disease, but that notion is now strictly of historical interest.[5,17] The spread of AIDS in the general population has not matched the rate of spread in high risk segments of the population, such as homosexual men and intravenous drug abusers, but it has outpaced early expectations.[17-20] Methods for detecting the virus were developed years after the start of the epidemic, and techniques for disabling the virus have yet to be developed.[21-24] Knowledge of how the virus spread failed to produce measures that curtailed the spread of the virus.[22,23] The initial impression that AIDS is a highly lethal condition caused by an exceedingly changeable virus is, unfortunately, one of the few early impressions of AIDS that has survived protracted scrutiny.[5,6,17,25]

IMMUNODEFICIENCY AND THE NERVOUS SYSTEM

The immune system's management of the nervous system is distinct from its management of other organ systems.[14] The blood-brain barrier between the blood stream and central nervous system (CNS) tissue sequesters or excludes some components of the immune system. As a result, truly local immune problems may develop in the central nervous system when elements of the immune system inside or outside the CNS are attacked or disturbed.

AIDS may cause nervous system problems initially, terminally, or during the evolution of the disease. That HIV can enter and attack the nervous system is probably independent of its ability to disable the immune barriers that guard nerve tissues.[24] The disabled immune system allows the nervous system to be attacked by opportunistic infections, such as toxoplasmosis, cytomegalovirus, cryptococcosis, and nocardiosis, at the same time that HIV itself is damaging nervous system components. Infections are currently the most common problems faced by AIDS patients with neurologic symptoms, but the organisms causing lethal infections in the nervous system, such as *Toxoplasma gondii* and *Cryptococcus neoformans*, are not always the same as the ones causing lethal problems outside the nervous system, such as *Pneumocystis* pneumonia.[26–31] Even if patients with HIV infection do not develop opportunistic infections in the nervous system, they are still at risk for developing a subacute encephalitis or myelitis from HIV itself.[11,32,33] Those who do not succumb to the AIDS-associated opportunistic infections or the HIV-induced encephalitis may develop primary non-Hodgkin's brain lymphomas.[34–36]

Central nervous system lymphomas were relatively uncommon as primary brain and spinal cord tumors before the widespread dissemination of AIDS.[5,34,36] These lymphomas may result from viral infections that induce malignant transformations in lymphocytes sequestered in the nervous system, or they may arise from less direct effects of the virus causing AIDS. In either case, such lymphomas are usually difficult to detect until they are widespread in the nervous system and difficult to treat even if they are detected before they are widespread.

Any combinations of these neurologic problems may occur. The damaged immune system leaves the AIDS victim vulnerable to all of these problems even if one of them is successfully treated. The enormous spectrum of problems developing in the CNS of patients with AIDS has frustrated efforts to realize protracted survival after signs and symptoms of nervous system disease have appeared.

SIGNS AND SYMPTOMS OF NERVOUS SYSTEM DISEASE

The neurologic signs and symptoms that evolve with AIDS are determined by what agent damages the nervous system, how severely damaged the nervous system is by the insult, and what locations in the nervous system are affected.[10,31,37] Equally important is the maturity of the nervous system. An adult with AIDS may develop generalized seizures evoked by a bacterial or fungal meningitis.[13] The infant with AIDS may exhibit profound developmental delays caused by prenatal infection.[32]

The nature of the injurious agent is often less important than the location of the injury. Patients are as likely to have focal weakness or seizures if the brain lesions associated with their AIDS infection is caused by either a fungal infection or a lymphoma. The same infection or tumor can cause different manifestations when distributed differently in the nervous system. Focal *Toxoplasma gondii* lesions may produce a hemiplegia, whereas widespread disease may produce dementia.[30,38] That the patient has signs and symptoms characteristic of nervous system damage is helpful in determining the best approach to investigating the patient's acute disease. However, what neurologic signs and symptoms develop with AIDS are of little help in identifying the specific causes of the acute changes.

THE BASIS FOR THE ACQUIRED IMMUNE DEFICIENCY SYNDROME

At a cellular level, the most distinctive feature of the immunodeficiency associated with AIDS is the depletion of a specific class of lymphocytes, the helper-inducer lymphocytes.[39–41] These are presumed to have matured in the thymus and are, therefore, called T-lymphocytes. T-lymphocytes help in the activation of several different components of the immune reaction to invading organisms and induce destructive actions by other cells in the immune system.[42] These helper-inducer lymphocytes, the principal targets of HIV, are designated in a variety of ways including T4, T4+, OKT4+, and CD4. The most popular designations are T4 and CD4.[3] All of these designations refer to a surface antigen, the T4 or CD4 antigen, with which this lymphocyte's cell membrane is replete. This family of lymphocytes interacts directly or indirectly with monocytes, macrophages, cytotoxic T cells, natural killer cells, B lymphocytes, and other vital elements of the immune system.[40] Without the CD4 T lymphocyte, much of the immune defense against intracellular and other types of infections fails.

The T4 (CD4) antigen, which can be detected with monoclonal antibodies that bind to it, constitutes part or all of the binding site for the human immunodeficiency virus.[8,43,44] Monoclonal antibodies have been used to identify other subtypes of T

lymphocytes, including the suppressor or CD8 (T8) lymphocyte, a subtype that normally occurs half as often as the CD4 subtype in the total lymphocyte population. In normal individuals, the ratio of CD4 T lymphocytes to CD8 T lymphocytes, CD4/CD8 (T4/T8), in any volume of peripheral blood is greater than 2.0 but is characteristically decreased in patients with AIDS.

To infect T4 lymphocytes, the virus binds at the T4 antigen site. Other cells have this T4 (CD4) binding site, but none has as many per unit of cell surface as the helper-inducer T lymphocyte. CD4 receptors or similar structures are probably present on some of the nervous system cells that are attacked by the virus, but damage to the nervous system is too extensive to be explained by the few antigenic sites that have been detected.[44] Indeed, much of the damage inflicted on lymphocytes, macrophages, and cells in the nervous system is not necessarily from direct attack by HIV at all. Abnormal secretions, changes in cell membrane characteristics, and disturbed cell activities may allow one infected cell to injure or kill many other cells that are not directly infected.

HIV does not cause disease as soon as it is acquired and, in fact, may require a specific change in the cell it has infected or a change in the environment of that cell before it becomes active. This may account for the apparent predilection of human immunodeficiency virus for the nervous system even in individuals without the full-blown immunodeficiency syndrome. The immunologic characteristics of the central nervous system may allow activation of the virus before infected cells on the other side of the blood-brain barrier are stimulated to trigger viral replication.

Monocytes and at least some of the macrophages that differentiate from monocytes have the CD4 marker on their surfaces and become infected with HIV.[8,40] One of the many questions raised by the central nervous system infection with HIV is how the virus gets past the barriers preventing other infections from entering this closed system. Some investigators believe that infected monocytes migrate across the blood-brain barrier, carrying with them and later releasing the human immunodeficiency virus into the central nervous system.[45,46] In patients with AIDS and evidence of the virus in the central nervous system, most of the HIV material that can be identified is found in monocytes and macrophages.

Immune System Problems

Much remains to be understood about the effects of HIV. The lymphocytes infected with the virus usually are killed during viral replication, but how this occurs and why it does not invariably occur are still unknown.[6,40] Patients with AIDS typically have T4 (CD4) lymphocyte counts of less than 200 to 400 cells/μL.[3,47] Other families of lymphocytes may be largely unaffected or depleted to a lesser degree. Part of CD4 lymphocyte depletion may actually be a response of the intact components of the immune system. Specialized T lymphocytes, called killer cells, attack other lymphocytes and macrophages infected with the virus.[48] Even if this destructive interaction does not contribute substantially to the weakening of the immune system, it may produce counterproductive inflammatory reactions in organs like the brain and lung, which subsequently develop opportunistic infections.[48]

Disturbed immune system function is manifested in several ways in patients with AIDS. Defects in cell-mediated immunity allow specific types of infections usually held in check by cell-mediated immunity to occur. Esophageal candidiasis and *Pneumocystic carinii* pneumonia are especially prevalent in affected patients.[49] Infection with fungi other than *Candida* organisms, such as cryptococci, also occur and frequently involve the central nervous system.[31] *Toxoplasma gondii*, an obligate in-

tracellular protozoan, affects other organs, but it is especially damaging and aggressive in the central nervous system.[30]

More pathogenic organisms also find the patient with AIDS an easy target. Nontuberculous, as well as tuberculous, mycobacteria may cause systemic or CNS infections. Herpes zoster, herpes simplex, and cytomegalovirus eruptions or disseminated infections may develop. Presumably the patient carries these viruses in a latent form until the immune deficiency allows them to become active.

Additional immune system problems that develop with AIDS include inappropriate production of autoantibodies, immune complex formation, and tissue injury.[39] This has special relevance for the nervous system since some of the autoantibodies produced cause thrombocytopenia and increase the risk of intracerebral and subarachnoid hemorrhage.[50,51] Patients with AIDS have unsuppressed or inappropriate immunoglobulin synthesis, which results in a characteristic hypergammaglobulinemia.[39] This may contribute to the development of peripheral neuropathies in many of the AIDS patients who develop idiopathic neuropathies.

Human Immunodeficiency Viruses (HIV)

Although more than one distinct virus causes AIDS, they are all similar in structure and behavior and are grouped in the family of human immunodeficiency viruses (HIV).[52,53] This virus has been called human T-cell lymphotropic virus-type III (HTLV-III), lymphadenopathy-associated virus (LAV), and the AIDS-associated retrovirus (ARV). Its current designation as the human immunodeficiency virus (HIV) reflects the consensus that this is an infectious agent, which is especially lethal for elements of the immune system of one species, *Homo sapiens*.[53,54]

Human immunodeficiency virus (HIV) belongs to a large family of viruses called retroviruses. Typical of retroviruses is that they contain two identical strands of RNA in their core, as well as copies of a protein, reverse transcriptase (Plate 1-1). This transcriptase enzyme initiates translation of the viral RNA into a DNA message after a host cell has been invaded. The specific group of retroviruses that HIV most resembles are the lentiviruses, retroviruses with an affinity for the nervous system, as well as other organ systems, and with a proclivity to kill cells that they infect.[55–57] (Table 1-1) HIV is the first lentivirus recognized to infect humans and cause disease.

Previously studied lentiviruses often caused neurologic diseases characterized by subacute encephalopathies. In many ways, including this capacity to cause a subacute encephalitis, HIV has proven to be similar to its fellow lentiviruses. In fact, in terms of structure and function, HIV is very similar to a lentivirus causing an AIDS-like disease in macaque monkeys in Africa.[58,59] This simian immunodeficiency virus (SIV) or STLV-III causes immune system damage and a subacute encephalitis in nonhuman primates and may be derived from the same virus that gave rise to HIV.

Characteristic of lentiviruses is their tendency to have protracted delays between acquisition and expression of disease and to produce latent or persistent disease.[57,60] They also exhibit restricted viral gene expression and a remarkable degree of genomic variation.[60] Not all of the genes coded by the virus are activated when a cell is infected. Instead much of the genetic material encoded by the virus regulates the expression of other viral genes. The genomic variation observed in lentiviruses results in numerous distinct strains of each type of lentivirus, a feature that complicates the production of an effective vaccine. Visna, a lentivirus that causes subacute encephalitis in sheep, and SIV, the lentivirus that infects macaque monkeys, also produce pathologic changes in the brain, but these are different from the pathology caused by HIV infection in the human central nervous system.

STRUCTURE OF HIV

Every human immunodeficiency virus consists of little more than a string of ribonucleic acid (RNA) enclosed in a glycoprotein coat.[54,61] All of the information needed for replication of the virus is encoded in the core ribonucleic acid chain. No deoxyribonucleic acid (DNA), the molecule used for genetic information storage by all true cells, is present in this virus. The glycoprotein coat or envelope surrounding the viral RNA core is essential for attaching to and entering cells.[53] This envelope around the viral core consists of two glycoproteins, one weighing 120 kilodaltons and the other weighing 41 kilodaltons, the heavier glycoprotein facing out of the coat membrane and the lighter facing in[62] (Fig. 1-1). These envelope glycoproteins are called gp120 and gp41.[53,63]

Packaged along with the RNA in the virus core is a protein, reverse transcriptase, which initiates the complex chain of genetic events that enables the viral RNA to be translated into a readable DNA message.

Table 1-1. Lentiviruses which Attack the Central Nervous System

Host	Retrovirus	Common Features
Man	Human immunodeficiency virus	Prolonged incubation period
Monkey	Simian immunodeficiency virus	Persistent or latent infection
Sheep	Visna virus	Restricted viral gene expression
Horses	Equine infectious anemia virus	Subacute encephalitis induced
Goats	Caprine arthritis encephalitis virus	Genomic variation

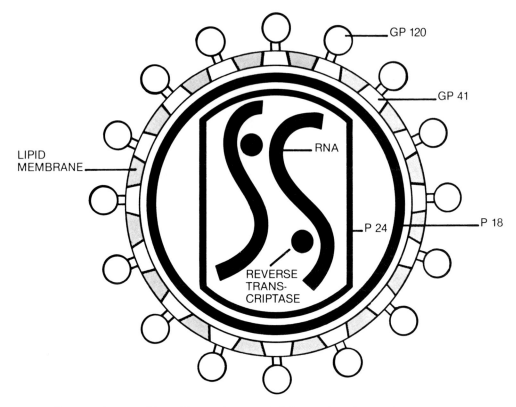

Fig. 1-1. Structural composition of human immunodeficiency virus (HIV), the retrovirus that causes AIDS. The most superficial protein constituent of the viral envelope is the glycoprotein gp120. Facing inward is gp41 glycoprotein, which extends through the lipid membrane of the viral envelope. The core protein p18 is more superficial than p24.

Before new viral particles can be created, the virus must enter a living cell and commandeer the cell's protein factories. The glycoprotein coat is essential to the invasion of the cell, and the transcriptase enzyme is essential to starting the process of viral takeover of the cell's production equipment.

Along with RNA and transcriptase, there are proteins in the core of the complete virus or virion. Two of the major proteins weigh 17 to 18 kilodaltons and 24 kilodaltons and are called p17 or p18 and p24 respectively. These core proteins are completely covered by the lipid and glycoprotein envelope that surrounds the core and can be detected in vitro only by

lysing the virion. Patients with HIV infection may produce antibodies to them, but these are not as easily measured as the antibodies produced against the various components of the viral envelope.

HIV REPLICATION

HIV is classified as a retrovirus because it reverses the usual process of DNA transcription into RNA.[54,61,64] All human cells transcribe the genetic information coded in their DNA into RNA and translate much of the RNA into proteins. In the normal multiplication of human cells, copies of the nuclear DNA are created as part of the process of cell division. Replication of an RNA virus must use distinctly different pathways, even though it is largely dependent upon what it finds in the cell it infects (see Plate 1-2).

The reverse transcriptase brought into the infected cell by the virus is an RNA-dependent DNA polymerase: It transcribes the viral RNA message into a string of DNA nucleotides.[61,65] The viral reverse transcriptase uses the infected cell's nucleotides to construct the DNA version of the RNA virus.[54,66] Once this DNA version, called a provirus, of the viral genetic material has been formed, the genetic code of the retrovirus can reproduce itself, direct the manufacture of viral structural elements, or simply persist in the infected cell.[54,65,67] The cell's machinery for interpreting DNA will blindly generate RNA and viral proteins based on the instructions encoded in the retrovirus-based DNA chain.[66] What determines whether the virus lies dormant in the cell for years or immediately begins replication is unknown. Nor is it known what determines when the infected cell dies and whether it necessarily dies prematurely.

HIV STRAINS

The exact structure of the HIV envelope varies from country to country and even from individual to individual. Although all human immunodeficiency viruses will lyse cells that they infect in culture and have a marked predilection for lymphoid cells, they are not immunologically identical.[65,68] This structural diversity caused confusion when the virus was originally detected. Some investigators included it in the family of human T-cell lymphotropic viruses (HTLVs), a group of closely related retroviruses, some of which are believed to cause progressive spinal cord damage.[7,21,33,69,70] A separate family of human immunodeficiency viruses was established when it was apparent that the composition and behavior of this AIDS-producing virus was distinctly different from HTLVs and justified its inclusion with the lentivirus subfamily of retroviruses.[56]

There are at least two distinct human immunodeficiency viruses (HIVs), each of which exhibits considerable variability from strain to strain.[6,52,59,71] These have been designated HIV-1 and HIV-2. HIV-1, the virus first discovered to cause AIDS, is widespread throughout the United States, Europe, and central Africa. It probably arose from HIV-2, a strain less virulent and more closely related to other primate retroviruses, including the simian immunodeficiency virus (SIV) of macaque monkeys.[72] HIV-2 is found primarily in Africa.[52,59]

Precipitating Factors

Genetic factors in individuals exposed to HIV may affect susceptibility to AIDS, but this is very controversial.[73] Some investigators claim that vulnerability to AIDS correlates with the presence or absence of group-specific component proteins (Gc), cell surface proteins that occur in one of six combinations of three subtypes.[73] Gc is involved in calcium transport across the cell membrane and may regulate viral entry into cells that become infected. The three major subtypes of Gc are 1 slow (1s), 1 fast (1f), and 2.[74] All are produced by a gene on chromosome 4, and each individual has two subtypes expressed according to the genes inherited from one's parents.

According to some investigators, individuals with a double dose of Gc 2 have the least risk of developing AIDS.[73] Those with a double dose of Gc 1f are at greatest risk of developing AIDS on exposure to HIV. Other combinations of Gc subtypes less clearly affect susceptibility or resistance. Population studies indicate that central African blacks have a higher incidence of susceptible subtypes than British or American whites.[73] There is no substantial difference between homosexual and heterosexual populations in terms of the distribution of these subtypes. The principal difference in the structure of the protein subtypes appears to be the number of sialic acid moieties attached. Patients with Gc 1f and high risk have two sialic acid moieties; those with Gc 2 and low risk have no sialic acid moieties attached to the Gc protein.

The sialic acid may facilitate attachment of HIV to cell surfaces. Homosexual men who have not developed antibodies to HIV despite repeated exposure to HIV infected partners most often have the Gc 2 variant.[73] Regions in Africa with a high incidence of AIDS have a high incidence of the double Gc 1f subtype in the population. This genetic difference might help explain why AIDS spread much more quickly in heterosexual communities in Africa than in England or the United States.

Investigators in the United States dispute this association between susceptibility to AIDS and Gc subtypes in homosexual populations, but they can identify individuals routinely exposed to the virus by virtue of their sexual practices who have not developed AIDS.[74,75] If Gc protein subtypes are not the basis for this apparent resistance to AIDS, another factor may be responsible. The most obvious explanation is that the resistance is more apparent than real. The patients who appear resistant to the infection may actually have the virus but are slow to produce antibodies to the virus. Until recently, population studies on the transmission of AIDS have relied on finding antibodies to the virus in the blood of victims, rather than on finding HIV antigens.[50]

In some patients, preexisting infection with other viruses may increase the probability of developing AIDS when infection with HIV occurs. Human T-cell lymphotropic virus I (HTLV-I) does not cause AIDS, but patients with HTLV-I infection who subsequently develop HIV infection appear to have a much more rapid deterioration than patients with HIV infection alone. The enhancement of disease with preexisting retrovirus infection suggests that the initial virus may act as a catalyst or cofactor in infection.

AIDS-Related Complex (ARC)

Patients with premonitory signs of AIDS, but without the full immunodeficiency syndrome, generally have been designated as having an AIDS-related complex (ARC). This designation was important before the identification of HIV as the agent responsible for AIDS, but it is becoming of strictly historical interest. Before the pathophysiology of AIDS was at all understood, the signs and symptoms of ARC helped to identify individuals at high risk of developing AIDS. Risk of developing AIDS is now established by identifying HIV or HIV antigens in the patient and measuring lymphocyte depletion or other hematologic changes produced by HIV infection.[3,50,76]

Problems typically exhibited by patients classified as having an AIDS-related complex (ARC) include both clinical and laboratory abnormalities (Table 1-2).[77] Two clinical abnormalities in association with two hematologic abnormalities generally establish that an individual has ARC. The clinical criteria include unexplained weight loss in excess of 10 percent of customary body weight, unexplained fevers over the course of 3 or more months, lymphadenopathy lasting more than 3 months, unexplained diarrhea, night sweats, and chronic

Table 1-2. Problems Typical of AIDS-Related Complex

Clinical	Laboratory
Weight loss	Reduced helper-inducer T
Diarrhea	cells
Fever	Diminished helper/suppressor
Night sweats	ratio
Lymphadenopathy	Decreased
Oral hairy	lymphoproliferative
leukoplakia	responses
Oral candidiasis	Increased polyclonal gamma
Herpes zoster	globulins

fatigue.[78] Many of these patients also have herpes zoster lesions and oral hairy leukoplakia.[47] The hematologic abnormalities considered diagnostic of ARC include depression of the CD4 (helper-inducer) T lymphocyte count, reduction of the helper/suppressor lymphocyte ratio to less than 1.0, decreased lymphoproliferative responses, and increased serum globulins.[77]

These criteria are fairly stringent and have never been universally applied. Some investigators accept the diagnosis of ARC if the patient has at least two of the following: (1) fatigue or diarrhea or oral temperature in excess of 37.8°C lasting 2 or more weeks, (2) unintentional weight loss of more than 4.5 kg over a 6-month interval, and (3) potassium-hydroxide confirmed oral thrush.[79]

Future designations of patients at risk of developing AIDS will presumably rely exclusively on hematologic parameters that correlate with impending deterioration of the immune system.[76] The patient with antibodies to HIV and a CD4 T lymphocyte count of less than 250 cells/μL is more clearly at high risk of developing the full-blown acquired immunodeficiency syndrome than patients who meet the various criteria proposed for defining the AIDS-related complexes.[76] In studies done on hemophiliacs, the risk factors for developing AIDS do not include depression of the CD4 (T4) T lymphocyte count but do consistently include thrombocytopenia, HIV antigenemia, and low titers of core protein p24 antibodies.[50,80] As more specific viral antigens are measured and more restricted hematologic reactions to HIV are followed, the criteria for identifying individuals at risk for immunodeficiency or neurologic disease associated with HIV infection will become more accurate.

Incubation Period

The delay from acquisition of the virus to the appearance of AIDS has been estimated by observations on patients with ARC and those with single episodes of exposure to the virus, such as occurs with the transfusion of infected blood.[81] This is called the incubation period, but it is more accurately viewed as a dormant interval or latent period. Patients have the virus but have no substantial evidence of viral activity. After acquisition of the virus there may be a delay of weeks or months before the patient has detectable antibodies to any viral elements and a delay of weeks, months, or years before the patient exhibits progressive immunologic or neurologic disease.[50]

In children less than 5 years of age, the average interval before the appearance of AIDS from the day of acquisition of HIV is about 2 years. In many young patients, symptoms of immunodeficiency or neurologic disease appear 6 months to 2 years after infection with HIV, but several patients with incubation periods of over 5 years have been reported.[82] These children may not have met the criteria for the diagnosis of AIDS that existed at the time they first began to exhibit symptoms of HIV infection. What constitutes AIDS has been revised several times since the syndrome was originally described; thus, the actual interval from the time the child acquired the virus until the child had a disease that met the existing criteria for AIDS may have been artificially protracted. Many children may have had substantial damage attributable to HIV infection that was simply not considered sufficient to justify the diagnosis of AIDS.[82]

Even when the changing definition of AIDS is taken into consideration, the apparent latent period is surprisingly long in patients infected after infancy. Between 5 and 59 years of age, this average dormant interval extends to 8 years, and over the age of 60, it shortens to about 5.5 years.[81] These are extraordinarily long incubation periods and are based on mathematical projections, but case reports each month support the grim results predicted by these projections.[50,51] Patients who received transfusions in 1980 are still at risk of developing AIDS.

During this period of incubation, the virus is not necessarily entirely dormant. Strains of HIV that appear to be incapable of causing AIDS may still reproduce and infect nervous system cells.[6] These nonlethal variants could cause progressive dementia or neuropathy independent of immunodeficiency.

Not all people with HIV infections will necessarily develop AIDS, but what proportion will not is still unknown. Because the projected incubation periods may be several years and the epidemic has been critically studied for so few years, it is probable that most people with HIV infection will develop AIDS.[80] In fact, it is still possible, though not likely considering the experience with other lethal viral diseases, that every person with detectable HIV will eventually develop AIDS, and many of them will have profound dementia even before the full-blown syndrome appears.

DIAGNOSING AIDS

Patients with neurologic disease who are believed or known to harbor HIV pose two diagnostic problems: the establishment of the diagnosis of AIDS and the determination of the cause of the neurologic signs and symptoms. Establishing the diagnosis of AIDS still depends primarily on the appearance of nonneurologic signs of disease (Table 1-3). Most of these signs are amplifications of those used to establish a patient as at risk for AIDS. Patients need not exhibit all of these findings to be diagnosed as having AIDS, but most will exhibit several clinical and laboratory findings consistent with immunodeficiency simultaneously.[3]

Detecting and managing the infections that develop in the nervous system present innumerable problems that were rarely encountered before the start of the AIDS epidemic.[7,17,21] Without rapid and effective di-

Table 1-3. Common Nonneurologic Signs and Symptoms in AIDS

Clinical	Laboratory
Persistent lymphadenopathy	CD4 T-lymphocyte count below 400/μL
Fungus-like skin lesions	CD8 T-lymphocyte count above 1,200/μL
Weight loss in excess of 4.5 kg	CD4/CD8 ratio less than 0.9
Fatigue	Platelet count less than 150,000/μL
Diarrhea	Hematocrit less than 30%
Thrush	Neutrophil count less than 1,800/μL
	Polyclonal gamma globulinemia

agnosis and treatment, patients with AIDS and nervous system disease invariably die.[31] Arriving at the correct diagnosis and instituting effective treatment is complicated by the lethal character of the responsible virus. In investigating the patient with AIDS, precautions must be taken to protect the patient from rapidly evolving complications and to protect involved medical personnel from contamination. Precautions must be taken in handling the fluids and tissues sampled as part of the routine investigation of the problem.[83–85] If a brain biopsy is necessary to characterize a mass or degenerative process, the neurosurgical technique must be tailored to minimize the risk of spreading the virus.

Diagnostic Modalities

With the development of assays for measuring antibodies to and antigens in the human immunodeficiency viruses, individuals who have been exposed to the virus can be identified. Widely used techniques include the enzyme-linked immunosorbent assay (ELISA) and the Western blot method.[78] Radioimmunoprecipitation techniques of varying complexity have also been useful in identifying individuals who have been exposed to HIV.[62]

The most widely used screening test is

the ELISA test for HIV antibody.[9,86] The antibodies measured are primarily those formed against the viral envelope glycoproteins.[62,87] The presence of antibodies to envelope glycoproteins does not mean that an individual has AIDS. It simply indicates an immune reaction to the virus and, therefore, exposure to the virus.

The ELISA is performed several different ways, but the basic format is to add material, such as serum or CSF, that is being analyzed for antibodies to HIV to a small chamber with antibodies that will bind these HIV antibodies. This complex is then labeled by adding additional antibodies, which are linked directly or indirectly to an enzyme. The enzyme chosen is one that will produce a color change in solution when its substrate is added (Fig. 1-2).

In most facilities, positive ELISA tests are checked for accuracy by performing a more costly and time-consuming immunoblot analysis.[78,88] One version of this is the Western blot technique, an electrophoretic procedure in which the virus is lysed and

fractionated on a nitrosecellulose column.[78] Serum from the patient is applied to this strip of fractionated viral antigens; and, if antibodies to a core protein, such as p24, bind to the lysed viral components, they can be detected. False-positive results are much less likely with this technique than with the ELISA. More recently, direct detection of viral antigens, rather than antibodies to these antigens, has been used to establish the diagnosis of HIV, but this is still too complicated and expensive for wide application.[50]

An alternative to identification of a viral antigen, such as a core protein or envelope glycoprotein, is recovery of the viral genome from patients with suspected infections.[32,62] A solid-phase enzyme immunoassay has also been used to detect viral antigen in patients with neurologic signs of AIDS, but this is an exceedingly costly procedure.[32,88] Because of its low cost and simplicity, the ELISA test will continue to be the primary testing modality for HIV infection for several years.

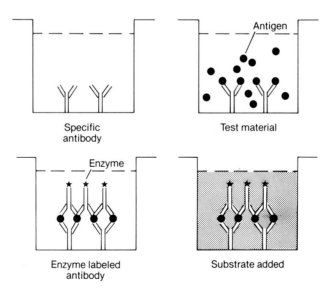

Fig. 1-2. Schematic of the ELISA test. Antibody to human anti-HIV antibody coats the bottom of wells on test plates. If material is added to the wells containing anti-HIV antibodies, those antibodies will be bound in the well. Adding immunoglobulins linked to an enzyme allows detection of the anti-HIV when the substrate for the enzyme is added.

That the patient has antibodies to HIV or HIV antigens retrievable from body fluids or tissues does not mean that the patient has the acquired immunodeficiency syndrome. Individuals can carry the virus for months or years without developing AIDS.[79] Rare individuals may even be able to contain the infection permanently and never develop AIDS, but prospective studies have been conducted for too short a time to establish this possibility. The earliest signs of progressive immunodeficiency in the patient with HIV infection appear to be a declining number of CD4 (T4+) T lymphocytes in the peripheral blood or an increase in the level of HIV antigen in the serum.[50,79] The fall in CD4 T lymphocytes to less than 250 cells/μL is often, but not always, reflected in a reduction in the total number of lymphocytes to under 1,000/μL.[39]

Several techniques available for measuring the ratio of CD4 (helper-inducer) T lymphocytes to CD8 (suppressor-cytotoxic) T lymphocytes in peripheral blood may be as useful as detecting a fall in the absolute number of CD4 T lymphocytes.[39,89] Normally the ratio of these lymphocyte populations is 2.0 (CD4/CD8).[39,89] A ratio of less than 0.9 to 1.0 is generally considered consistent with AIDS.[89]

The patient's inability to resist opportunistic infections in AIDS is reflected in an inability to respond to standard tests of immune function, such as anergy panels. The victim of AIDS does not respond to commonly occurring antigens, such as trichophyton, candida, tetanus toxoid, and purified protein derivative. Although the anergy panel is very nonspecific, it is also extremely inexpensive and simple to perform.

Confidence Limits

All of the tests currently available to diagnose AIDS have limitations. HIV infection can be most confidently diagnosed if the virus is isolated and cultured from the patient, but viral cultures on every suspected carrier are impractical, because of their cost and complexity. Checking for antibodies to HIV in the serum is relatively simple, but false-positive and false-negative tests are unavoidable with any screening technique.[86] Complicating matters further is the discovery that seroconversion may be delayed for weeks or months after the virus is actively replicating in an individual.[9] Because AIDS may spread through the use of tainted blood and infected organs, the prospect of virus-positive, but antibody-negative, material is complicating medical management enormously. The probability of such material being reponsible for infection is exceedingly low, but as the population of HIV infected individuals increases the absolute number of such transmissions will increase.

INDICATOR DISEASES

Some diseases are so unlikely in the absence of AIDS that they have been adopted as circumstantial evidence of the syndrome.[3] Such indicator diseases include candidiasis of the esophagus, trachea, bronchi, or lungs; extrapulmonary cryptococosis; protracted cryptosporidiosis with diarrhea; Kaposi's sarcoma in a patient less than 60 years of age; lymphoid interstitial pneumonia or pulmonary lymphoid hyperplasia in a patient less than 13 years of age; *Pneumocystic carinii* pneumonia; and disseminated *Mycobacterium avium* complex (Table 1-4). Several problems specifically affecting the nervous system are considered indicator diseases.[3] These include cytomegalovirus infection in the CNS in a patient older than 1 month of age, primary brain lymphoma in a patient less than 60 years of age, cerebral toxoplasmosis in a patient over 1 month of age, and progressive multifocal leukoencephalopathy in a patient

Table 1-4. Indicator Diseases

Adults	Children	Adults and Children
Kaposi's sarcoma	Lymphoid interstitial pneumonia	Primary brain lymphoma
Cytomegalovirus encephalitis	Pulmonary lymphoid hyperplasia	*Pneumocystis carinii* pneumonia
Cerebral toxoplasmosis		Candidiasis of the oropharynx or lungs
		Extrapulmonary cryptococcosis
		Cryptosporidiosis with diarrhea
		Disseminated *Mycobacterium avium* complex
		Progressive multifocal leukoencephalopathy

with no other apparent predisposing conditions.[3]

If patients exhibit any of these problems, they probably have AIDS unless they have been on long-term immunosuppressant therapy of some sort within 3 months of developing the indicator disease or they have another condition that will necessarily interfere with immune function. Immune disorders routinely occur with Hodgkin's disease, non-Hodgkin's lymphomas, lymphocytic leukemias, multiple myeloma, angioimmunoblastic lymphadenopathy, and other lymphoreticular or histiocytic malignancies.[3] Rare individuals have congenital immunodeficiency syndromes or even acquired syndromes unrelated to HIV infection, but these are usually adequately distinctive to cause no confusion.[3]

COMPLICATING FACTORS

Even if an individual has one of these immune system depressing problems, current evidence favors the diagnosis of AIDS if an indicator disease develops along with laboratory evidence of HIV infection.[3] People with systemic lymphomas or Hodgkin's disease may contract the human immunodeficiency virus and develop *Pneumocystis carinii* pneumonia, in which case they are lymphoma victims with AIDS.[3] With laboratory evidence of HIV infection, the appearance of any one of several typical problems is diagnostic of AIDS.[3] These typical

problems include intractable emaciation, recurrent nontyphoidal *Salmonella* septicemia, extrapulmonary tuberculosis, nontuberculous mycobacterial disease, several types of non-Hodgkin's lymphomas, protracted isosporiasis with diarrhea, disseminated histoplasmosis, disseminated coccidioidomycosis, and a variety of recurrent bacterial infections in children.[3]

Finding evidence of HIV infection, such as antibodies in the serum or cerebrospinal fluid or isolation of the virus from any tissue, is important in confidently making the diagnosis of AIDS, but some patients will have indicator diseases and no other substantial basis for the diagnosis.[3] Reinforcing the conclusion that these patients do have AIDS is the finding of a T4 (CD4) lymphocyte count of less than 250 cells/μL.

Precautions

The investigation of patients with AIDS presents its own problems for the physicians and ancillary staff involved in the studies. This is a contagious disease that is certainly transmissible through blood and other fluids handled during a routine investigation.[4] All individuals handling potentially infectious tissues must avoid direct contact with the materials.

As part of the neurologic investigation, blood, spinal fluid, and brain tissue are all likely to be collected and processed. Brain biopsy is especially valuable in managing central nervous system complications of AIDS. Intact virus is easily isolated from brain and spinal cord tissues, so rigorous precautions must be taken in handling the tissues.[4] Neurosurgeons directly involved in handling brain tissue and body fluids should use double gloves.[35] A Mackenzie perforator, rather than an air drill, will reduce dispersal of material from the operative site when burr holes are created.[35] The bone plate removed to create a window through which the biopsy can be performed may be created with a Gigli saw.[35] If stereotactic techniques are feasible, they should be used so that a bone window need not be made. All specimens and blood should be placed in specially labeled containers so that any accidents that may occur during processing will be managed with special care.[4]

EVOLVING DEFINITIONS OF AIDS

Since the existence of AIDS was first suspected, the evolution of its definition has led to an increasingly diverse population of AIDS victims. This distorts comparisons of disease incidence figures over the past decade, but it reinforces the growing consensus that much that was not recognized as acquired immunodeficiency is AIDS as certainly as that defined by the most recent criteria.[3]

To an increasing extent, AIDS is being equated with progressive, disabling HIV infection, whether that infection is manifest as profound leukopenia and *Pneumocystis* pneumonia or as subacute encephalitis and progressive dementia. Also to an increasing extent AIDS is being recognized as a neurologic problem. Controlling opportunistic infections outside the central nervous system has not improved the outlook for individuals with problems in the central nervous system. Progressive encephalopathy is becoming as prominent a feature of HIV infection as immunodeficiency. Indeed,

with improved management of systemic infections and more effective antiviral agents suppressing the immune damage caused by the virus, the full impact of HIV on the central and peripheral nervous system may become evident. AIDS may soon be redefined as a syndrome in which reversible immunodeficiency is associated with progressive dementia, spasticity, ataxia, and seizures.

REFERENCES

1. Popovic M, Sarngadharan MG, Read E, Gallo RC: Detection, isolation, and continuous production of cytopathic retroviruses (HTLV-III) from patients with AIDS and pre-AIDS. Science 224:497, 1984
2. Levy JA, Hoffman AD, Kramer SM, et al: Isolation of lymphocytopathic retroviruses from San Francisco patients with AIDS. Science 225:840, 1984
3. CDC: Revision of the CDC surveillance case definition for acquired immunodeficiency syndrome. MMWR 36:3s, 1987
4. FDA: Special AIDS issue. FDA Drug Bull 17:14, 1987
5. CDC: Pneumocystis pneumonia—Los Angeles. MMWR 30:250, 1981
6. Anand R, Siegal F, Reed C, et al: Non-cytocidal natural variants of human immunodeficiency virus isolated from AIDS patients with neurological disorders. Lancet 2:234, 1987
7. Gallo RC, Sarin PS, Gelmann EP, et al: Isolation of human T-cell leukemia virus in acquired immune deficiency syndrome (AIDS). Science 220:865, 1983
8. Marx JL: The AIDS virus—well known but a mystery. Science 236:390, 1987
9. Landesman SH, Ginzburg HM, Weiss SH: The AIDS epidemic. N Engl J Med 312:521, 1985
10. Navia BA, Jordan BD, Price RW: The AIDS dementia complex: I. Clinical features. Ann Neurol 19:517, 1986
11. Navia BA, Price RW: The acquired immunodeficiency syndrome dementia complex as the presenting or sole manifestation of

human immunodeficiency virus infection. Arch Neurol 44:65, 1987

12. Vinters HV: The AIDS dementia complex. Ann Neurol 21:612, 1987
13. Harris AA, Segretti J, Levin S: Central nervous system infections in patients with the acquired immunodeficiency syndrome. Clin Neuropharmacol 8:201, 1985
14. Cotman CW, Brinton RE, Galaburda A, et al: The Neuro-Immune-Endocrine Connection. Raven Press, New York, 1987
15. Coffin J, Haase A, Levy JA, et al: Human immunodeficiency virus. Science 236:697, 1986
16. Anders KH, Guerra WF, Tomiyasu U, et al: The neuropathology of AIDS. UCLA experience and review. Am J Pathol 124:537, 1986
17. Centers for Disease Control Task Force on Kaposi's Sarcoma and Opportunistic Infections: Epidemiologic aspects of the current outbreak of Kaposi's sarcoma and opportunistic infections. N Engl J Med 306:248, 1982
18. Curran JW, Morgan WM, Hardy AM, et al: The epidemiology of AIDS: current status and future prospects. Science 229:1352, 1985
19. Hardy AM, Allen JR, Morgan WM, et al: The incidence rate of acquired immunodeficiency syndrome in selected populations. JAMA 253:215, 1985
20. Edwards DD: Heterosexuals and AIDS: mixed messages. Science News 132:60, 1987
21. Barré-Sinoussi F, Chermann J-C, Rey F, et al: Isolation of a T-lymphotropic retrovirus from a patient at risk for acquired immune deficiency syndrome (AIDS). Science 220:868, 1983
22. Curran J: The epidemiology and prevention of acquired immunodeficiency syndrome. Ann Intern Med 103:657, 1985
23. Coolfont report: a PHS plan for prevention and control of AIDS and the AIDS virus. Public Health Rep 101:341, 1986
24. Gallo RC, Salahuddin SZ, Popovic M, et al: Frequent detection and isolation of cytopathic retroviruses (HTLV-III) from patients with AIDS and at risk for AIDS. Science 224:500, 1984
25. Quinn TC, Mann JM, Curran JW, Piot P: AIDS in Africa: an epidemiologic paradigm. Science 234:955, 1986

26. Koppel BS, Wormser GP, Tuchman AJ, et al: Central nervous system involvement in patients with acquired immunodeficiency syndrome. Acta Neurol Scand 71:337, 1985
27. Herman P: Neurologic complications of acquired immunologic deficiency syndrome. Neurology 33:suppl. 2, 105, 1983
28. Levy RM, Pons VG, Rosenblum ML: Central nervous system mass lesions in the acquired immunodeficiency syndrome (AIDS). J Neurosurg 61:9, 1984
29. Wang B, Gold JWM, Brown AE, et al: Central-nervous-system toxoplasmosis in homosexual men and parenteral drug abusers. Ann Intern Med 100:36, 1984
30. Navia BA, Petito CK, Gold JWH, et al: Cerebral toxoplasmosis complicating AIDS: clinical and neuropathological findings in 27 patients. Ann Neurol 19:224, 1986
31. Levy RM, Bredesen DE, Rosenblum ML: Neurologic manifestations of the acquired immunodeficiency syndrome (AIDS): Experience at the University of California at San Francisco and review of the literature. J Neurosurg 62:475, 1985
32. Shaw GM, Harper ME, Hahn BH, et al: HTLV-III infection in brains of children and adults with AIDS encephalopathy. Science 227:177, 1985
33. Osame M, Matsumoto M, Usuku K, et al: Chronic progressive myelopathy associated with elevated antibodies to human T-lymphotropic virus type I and adult T-cell leukemialike cells. Ann Neurol 21:117, 1987
34. So YT, Beckstead HJ, Davis RL: Primary central nervous system lymphoma in acquired immune deficiency syndrome: a clinical and pathological study. Ann Neurol 20:566, 1986
35. Snow RB, Lavyne MH: Intracranial space-occupying lesions in acquired immunodeficiency syndrome patients. Neurosurg 16:148, 1985
36. Snider WD, Simpson DM, Aronyk KE, Nielsen SL: Primary lymphoma of the nervous system associated with acquired immune-deficiency syndrome. N Engl J Med 308:45, 1983
37. Navia BA, Jordan BD, Price RW: The AIDS dementia complex: II. Neuropathology. Ann Neurol 19:525, 1986
38. Farkash AE, Maccabee PJ, Sher JA, et al:

CNS toxoplasmosis in acquired immune deficiency syndrome: a clinical-pathological-radiological review of 12 cases. J Neurol Neurosurg Psychiatry 49:744, 1986

39. Shannon KM, Amman AJ: Acquired immune deficiency syndrome in childhood. J Pediatr 106:332, 1985

40. Ho DD, Pomerantz RJ, Kaplan JC: Pathogenesis of infection with human immunodeficiency virus. N Engl J Med 317:278, 1987

41. Kanki PJ, M'Boup S, Ricard D, et al: Human T-lymphotropic virus type 4 and the human immunodeficiency virus in West Africa. Science 236:827, 1987

42. Unanue ER, Allen PM: The basis for the immunoregulatory role of macrophages and other accessory cells. Science 236:551, 1987

43. Klatzmann D, Champagne E, Chamaret S, et al: T-lymphocyte T4 molecule behaves as receptor for human retroviral LAV. Nature 312:767, 1984

44. Maddon PJ, Dagleish AG, McDougal JS, et al: The T4 gene encodes the AIDS virus receptor and is expressed in the immune system and the brain. Cell 47:333, 1986

45. Koenig S, Gendelman HE, Orenstein JM, et al: Detection of AIDS virus in macrophages in brain tissue from AIDS patients with encephalopathy. Science 233:1089, 1986

46. Ho DD, Rota TR, Hirsch MS: Infection of monocyte/macrophages by human T lymphotropic virus type III. J Clin Invest 77:1712, 1986

47. Fischl MA, Richman DD, Grieco MH, et al: The efficacy of azidothymidine (AZT) in the treatment of patients with AIDS and AIDS-related complex. N Engl J Med 317:185, 1987

48. Edwards DD: Killer cells, MHC: factors in AIDS? Science News 132:52, 1987

49. Gottlieb MB, Schroff R, Schanker HM, et al: *Pneumocystis carinii* pneumonia and mucosal candidiasis in previously healthy homosexual men: evidence of a new acquired cellular immunodeficiency. N Engl J Med 305:1425, 1981

50. Allain J-P, Laurian Y, Paul DA, et al: Long-term evaluation of HIV antigen and antibodies to p24 and gp41 in patients with hemophilia. N Engl J Med 317:1114, 1987

51. Desforges J, Mark EJ: Case record 41-1987. N Engl J Med 317:946, 1987

52. Marx JL: Probing the AIDS virus and its relatives. Science 236:1523, 1987

53. Knight DM, Flomerfelt FA, Ghrayeb J: Expression of the art/trs protein of HIV and study of its role in viral envelope synthesis. Science 236:837, 1987

54. Gallo RC: The first human retrovirus. Sci Am 255:88, 1986

55. Gonda MA, Braun MJ, Clements JE, et al: Human T-cell lymphotropic virus type III shares sequence homology with a family of pathogenic lentiviruses. Proc Natl Acad Sci USA 49:307, 1987

56. Sonigo P, Alizon M, Staskus K, et al: Nucleotide sequence of the visna lentivirus: relationship to the AIDS virus. Cell 42:369, 1985

57. Johnson RT: Viral Infections of the Nervous System. Raven Press, New York, 1982

58. Letvin NL, Daniel MD, Sehgal PK, et al: Induction of AIDS-like disease in macaque monkeys with T-cell tropic retrovirus STLV-III. Science 230:71, 1985

59. Clavel F, Mansinho K, Chamaret S, et al: Human immunodeficiency virus type 2 infection associated with AIDS in West Africa. N Engl J Med 316:180, 1987

60. Haase AT: Pathogenesis of lentivirus infections. Nature 322:130, 1986

61. Varmus H: Reverse transcription. Sci Am 257:56, 1987

62. Barin F, McLane MF, Allan JS, et al: Virus envelope protein of HTLV-III represents major target antigen for antibodies in AIDS patients. Science 228:1094, 1985

63. Kowalski M, Potz J, Basiripour L, et al: Functional regions of the envelope glycoprotein of human immunodeficiency virus type 1. Science 237:1351, 1987

64. Feinberg MB, Jarrett RF, Aldovini A, et al: HTLV-III expression and production involve complex regulation at the levels of splicing and translation of viral RNA. Cell 46:807, 1986

65. Johnson RT, McArthur JC: Myelopathies and retroviral infections. Ann Neurol 21:113, 1987

66. Gelmann EP, Popovic M, Blayney D, et al: Proviral DNA of a retrovirus, human T-cell leukemia virus, in two patients with AIDS. Science 220:862, 1983

67. Callahan R, Chiu I-M, Wong JFH, et al: A

new class of endogenous human retroviral genome. Science 228:1208, 1985

68. Bowen DL, Lane HC, Fauci AS: Immunopathogenesis of the acquired immunodeficiency syndrome. Ann Intern Med 103:704, 1985

69. Vernant JC, Maurs L, Gessain A, et al: Endemic tropical spastic paraparesis associated with human T-Lymphotropic Virus type I: a clinical and seroepidemiological study of 25 cases. Ann Neurol 21:123, 1987

70. Rodgers-Johnsons P, Gajdusek DC, Morgan O StC, et al: HTLV-I and HTLV-III antibodies and tropical spastic paraparesis. Lancet 2:1247, 1985

71. Newmark P: Variations of AIDS relatives. Nature 326:548, 1987

72. Gnann JW, McCormick JB, Mitchell S, et al: Synthetic peptide immunoassay distinguishes HIV type 1 and HIV type 2 infections. Science 237:1346, 1987

73. Eales L-J, Nye KE, Parkin JM, et al: Association of different allelic forms of group specific component with susceptibility to and clinical manifestation of human immunodeficiency virus infection. Lancet 1:999, 1987

74. Thymann M, Dickmeiss E, Svejgaard A, et al: AIDS and the Gc protein. Lancet 1:1378, 1987

75. Gilles K, Louie L, Newman B, et al: Genetic susceptibility to AIDS: absence of an association with group-specific component (Gc). N Engl J Med 317:630, 1987

76. Kaslow RA, Phair JP, Freidman HB, et al: Infection with human immunodeficiency virus: clinical manifestations and their relationship to immune deficiency. Ann Intern Med 107:474, 1987

77. Krause RM: Koch's postulates and the search for the AIDS agent. Rev Infect Dis 6:270, 1984

78. Hirsch MS, Wormser GP, Schooley RT, et al: Risk of nosocomial infection with human

T-cell lymphotropic virus III (HTLV-III). N Engl J Med 312:1, 1985

79. Polk BF, Fox R, Brookmeyer R, et al: Predictors of the acquired immunodeficiency syndrome developing in a cohort of seropositive homosexual men. N Engl J Med 316:61, 1987

80. Hilgartner MW: AIDS and hemophilia. N Engl J Med 317:1153, 1987

81. May RM, Anderson RM: Transmission dynamics of HIV infection. Nature 326:137, 1987

82. Epstein LG, Sharer LR, Oleske JM, et al: Neurologic manifestations of human immunodeficiency virus infection in children. Pediatrics 78:678, 1986

83. CDC: Recommendations for preventing transmission of infection with human T-lymphotropic virus type III/lymphadenopathy-associated virus during invasive procedures. MMWR 35:221, 1986

84. CDC: Recommendations for preventing possible transmission of HTLV-III/LAV from tears. MMWR 34:533, 1985

85. CDC: Update: human immunodeficiency virus infections in health-care workers exposed to blood of infected patients. MMWR 36:285, 1987

86. Weiss SH, Goedert JJ, Sarngadharan MG, et al: Screening test for HTLV-III (AIDS agent) antibodies: specificity, sensitivity, and applications. JAMA 253:221, 1985

87. Allan JS, Coligan JE, Barin F, et al: Major glycoprotein antigens that induce antibodies in AIDS patients are encoded by HTLV-III. Science 228:1091, 1985

88. Epstein LG, Goudsmit J, Paul DA, et al: Expression of human immunodeficiency virus in cerebrospinal fluid of children with progressive encephalopathy. Ann Neurol 21:397, 1987

89. Gebel HM, Anderson JE, Gottschalk LR, Bray RA: Determination of helper-suppressor T-cell ratios. N Engl J Med 316:113, 1987

2

Epidemiology

In October, 1347, several ships with ill sailors docked in Sicily to resupply themselves. They came from the east with survivors of the battle of Kaffa, a city that had fallen to the Mongols after a brief seige. The Mongols had faced only minor resistance because the city had been struck by disease shortly after the seige had begun. Within days or weeks, all of the sailors and passengers on these ships had died. Throughout the harbor town and surrounding countryside, the lethal illness spread faster than the population could evacuate. Without any antecedent complaints, healthy people fell prostrate and died within hours or days. The victims were of all ages, classes, and religious beliefs. Everyone was at risk; no one recovered once stricken.

The population had many names for the bubonic plague that these ships had brought into the Sicilian port, but history has settled on the Black Death as the most appropriate name for this disease. It had probably been in Asia for centuries, but it was an entirely new experience for Europe. The highly lethal infection spread to much of the population between Sicily and Paris by the winter of 1348. Mortality statistics are poor for the 14th century, but most estimates put deaths directly attributable to bubonic plague in Europe at about 25 million over the next 2 years. The plague was carried by infested rats, and the rats did not disappear. Over the next five decades, recurrent outbreaks of bubonic plague killed tens of millions of people throughout Europe.

The acquired immune deficiency syndrome (AIDS) appeared with the abruptness of the bubonic plague and has exhibited the kind of relentless spread that terrorized earlier populations. In 1982, the reports of deaths attributable to failure of the immune system in previously healthy homosexual men and newly arriving Haitian immigrants could no longer be dismissed as a statistical illusion.[1-4] Within 1 year, acquired immunodeficiency was generally acknowledged to be a discrete syndrome.[5-8] By the end of 1983, a virus had been convincingly linked to the syndrome.[9,10] Sexual activity and blood contamination proved to be the major routes for spread of the disease.[11] No one suspected how rapidly it would spread.

In 1984, AIDS was responsible for 3,000 deaths in the United States. This increased to 5,000 in 1985 and 9,000 in 1986. The number of patients reported to have or have had AIDS in the United States exceeded 43,500 by the end of 1987, and of these more than 25,000 had died. The number of Americans who were seropositive for HIV antibodies and, therefore, at high risk of developing AIDS by the end of 1984 was estimated already to be greater than 400,000.[12] By the end of 1987, seropositivity was evident in more than 1 million Americans. The World Health Organization estimated in mid-1987 that 5 to 10 million people worldwide had been infected by HIV, at least one-third of whom would develop AIDS within a few years.[13] Deaths in Africa caused by AIDS had reached many thousands per year by 1987 and was expected to reach millions per year when the epidemic finally peaked.

Conservative estimates place the annual death toll at over 50,000 in the United States alone by 1991. This will be only a tenth of the toll attributable to cancer in the United States, but AIDS has a greater social impact than cancer. It is a disease affecting the sexually active and the newborn. Those most victimized by the disease are those mature enough to work, involved in building families, and engaged in the activities that maintain the fabric of society. Newborns with the disease place an enormous medical and financial burden on the whole society and compound the personal and social tragedy caused by AIDS.

HIGH RISK GROUPS

When AIDS was first recognized in the United States, it was believed to be a problem limited to a few homosexual communities and recently arriving Haitian immigrants.[6,14,15] The identification of these two groups as those largely, if not solely, at risk for developing AIDS was politically unfortunate. Neither group commanded much political influence or generated much public sympathy. Subsequent reports that the disease was spreading among intravenous drug abusers further retarded the mobilization of resources to investigate and combat the disease. Reports of heterosexual spread of the disease in central Africa were initially distrusted. By the time the ability of the disease to spread to the general public was recognized, AIDS was already widely disseminated.

Table 2-1. High Risk Groups

Children	Adults
Mothers had HIV infection during pregnancy	IV drug abusers
	Sexual partners of IV drug abusers
Hemophiliacs and other blood product recipients	Homosexual and bisexual men
	Blood product recipients
Sexually abused	Male and female prostitutes
	Sexual partners of hemophiliacs
	Central Africans

Intravenous Drug Abusers

Intravenous drug abusers remain at high risk of developing AIDS (Table 2-1). As of 1987, they accounted for over 70 percent of the cases of AIDS among heterosexual men and women.[16] The common practice of sharing hypodermic needles has facilitated rapid spread of the virus through injection.[16] In the 1970s and 1980s, intravenous drug abusers in large American cities routinely injected illicitly purchased drugs in facilities called shooting galleries. A shooting gallery usually consisted of a set of rooms in an abandoned building in which hypodermic syringes and needles were available. The needles and syringes most commonly used were those widely available for insulin self-injection. The addict would borrow or rent a needle and syringe for drug injection and return the needle and syringe to the gallery pool after self-injection. As a result, a single needle might be used for several thousand injections in several hundred people in a single month. Needles were used until they clogged or broke: they were never sterilized.

CASE HISTORY ONE

A 60-year-old man with a long history of intravenous drug abuse and alcoholism was admitted because of weakness, 15 pound weight loss over the preceding year, and difficulty swallowing. On examination he had a maculopapular rash on his chest, back, and palms. Thrush was evident in his mouth, and his liver was enlarged.

His chest x-ray revealed a unilateral nodular infiltrate. Bronchial lavage and biopsy established that he had *Pneumocystis carinii* infection. Oral cultures yielded *Candida albicans*. Liver biopsy revealed chronic alcoholic liver disease. He had leukopenia with a white blood cell count of 1,700 cells/μL.

Within a few days of admission the patient developed paraparesis. His spinal fluid contained 100 lymphocytes/μL. Cytologic examination of the cerebrospinal fluid did not suggest lymphoma initially, but subsequent examinations did reveal abnormal lymphocytes with at least one large cell interpreted as a lymphoblast. He had daily fever spikes of 104°F and became progressively less responsive. No infectious basis for the fever was evident. The patient became intractably comatose. Within 2 months of admission the patient died.

At autopsy, the patient was found to have the acquired immune deficiency syndrome. The immediate cause of death was a primary lymphoma of the central nervous system (Fig. 2-1). The tumor cells were large, noncleaved, and widely disseminated in the brain tissue and the leptomeninges. There was an especially dense accumulation of tumor cells with focal necrosis in the right frontal lobe.

This patient was at high risk of developing AIDS because of his history of intravenous drug abuse. As is often the case, the initial presentation was confused by his alcoholism and the myriad problems to which that

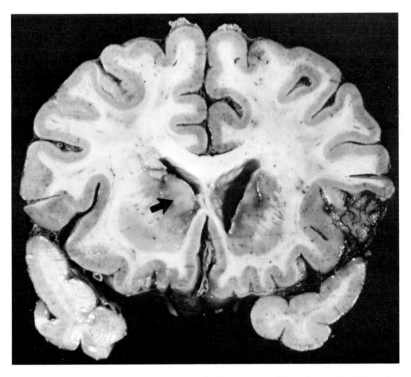

Fig. 2-1. Coronal section of the brain at the level of the rostral basal ganglia. The abnormal tissue in the caudate nuclei bilaterally represents primary brain lymphoma. This is most obvious on the left (arrow).

made him susceptible. Although he developed opportunistic infections as a consequence of his immune deficiency, it was a primary brain lymphoma that produced progressive neurologic deficits and death.

At least 200,000 of the estimated 750,000 intravenous drug abusers in the United States live in New York City.[17] Of these, more than 50 percent had antibodies to HIV by mid-1987.[17] In American urban centers, female prostitutes are often intravenous drug abusers who use prostitution to finance their drug addiction. As a result, women contracting AIDS through intravenous contamination provide the sexual transmission of the virus to heterosexual partners.[18]

Homosexual Men

Homosexual and bisexual men were among the first well-documented victims of AIDS and remain a group with extraordinarily high levels of HIV infection.[11,19–21] Random testing for HIV antibodies in large homosexual communities in New York City and San Francisco reveal exposure to and probable infection with HIV in more than 70 percent of the population.[16] An estimated 10 percent of the homosexual men in San Francisco have developed AIDS.[16] The rapid spread of the virus in these communities has been ascribed to a high level of promiscuity among homosexual men living in these cities, but this hypothesis has remained untested.

What is established is that homosexual and bisexual men are at increased risk of acquiring the syndrome if they have had repeated infections with syphilis, non-B hepatitis, or amebiasis and if they have highly diverse sexual practices.[20] The high level of anal intercourse practiced by this group has probably contributed more to the rapid spread of the disease than promiscuity per se. Studies in promiscuous women have failed to reveal any correlation between the probability of acquiring AIDS and the number of different sexual partners per week.[22] The type of sexual activity practiced by homosexual men, rather than promiscuity, appears to be the one trait specific to this group that could account for its susceptibility to AIDS.

Blood Product Recipients

Individuals who receive blood products frequently or regularly, such as individuals with hemophilia, are likely to develop antibodies to HIV.[23–26] As of the beginning of 1987, 2 percent of the adults and 12 percent of the children in the United States with AIDS acquired the infection through transfusions of blood or blood products that were tainted with HIV.[27] Precautions are extremely stringent to protect against the spread of HIV through blood or blood products, but measures to protect the 20,000 hemophiliacs in the United States alone and the tens of thousands of other individuals requiring blood transfusions were inadequate or unavailable before 1985. Since then, blood has been routinely checked for HIV antibodies and clotting factors are heat treated to inactivate undetected virus.[16,25]

Unfortunately, tens of thousands of people were probably exposed to HIV in blood products before these measures were widely available.[28,29] In the United States alone, at least 12,000 people were infected with HIV through blood or blood product transfusions before routine screening of blood for antibodies to HIV was instituted.[30,31] In adult hemophiliacs in the United States who received frequent transfusions between 1979 and 1987, the prevalence of antibodies against HIV ranges from 75 percent to 90 percent, and at least 20 percent of these hemophiliacs had developed AIDS or ARC by the end of 1987.[25] Children with hemophilia had a 58 percent prevalence of seroconversion and 4 percent to 5 percent of them had developed AIDS or ARC by the end of 1987.[25] The patients at special risk are those with hemophilia A or B. These patients were exposed to the virus if they received lyophilized concentrates, rather than cryoprecipitates, the important difference being that in the concentrates blood from thousands of donors is pooled.[31]

Sexual Partners of Carriers

The transmission of AIDS can occur through heterosexual intercourse.[32–34] As of June, 1987, 4 percent of the reported cases of AIDS were attributed to heterosexual activity with an infected partner.[22] Although a small component of the AIDS population, it is the fastest growing segment.[22] Of the more than 2,500 women in the United States who have had AIDS, at least 29 percent had no apparent exposure to the virus except during sexual intercourse with an infected man.[35] About 83 percent of the people acquiring AIDS through heterosexual activity are women.[16] Black and Hispanic women constitute the majority of women who have acquired AIDS through heterosexual activity.[22]

Most of the men in the United States who are infected have acquired the virus through homosexual activity, drug abuse, or transfusions. The most common of the unrecognized carriers is the bisexual man. This individual acquires the virus through homosexual activity and transmits it to women through heterosexual activity. The bisexual carrier need not be symptomatic for the disease to transmit it during heterosexual activity, but many will have a depressed number of CD4 (helper-inducer) T lymphocytes.[16]

At especially high risk are female sexual partners of men who apparently acquired AIDS through parenteral drug abuse.[8] Contact with only one sexual partner does not reduce the risk of acquiring the virus if that sexual partner is an infected drug addict. In 1982, 12 percent of the women with AIDS acquired it through heterosexual contact with men in high risk groups. By 1986 this had climbed to 26 percent of the women with AIDS.[36] It is now evident that transmission of the virus to women through strictly vaginal intercourse is common.

Children of HIV Infected Women

An increasing number of children contract AIDS each year.[37,38] In most cases, these children appear to acquire the disease from their mothers in utero.[31] Women with HIV infection often, and perhaps always, transmit the virus to their fetuses during development or at the time of birth. Clinical abnormalities in children who have acquired the virus by this route are usually apparent within a few months of birth.[31] These children have low birth weights and routinely exhibit hepatosplenomegaly; hence the virus is almost certainly acquired weeks or months before birth.[31] Caesarean section does not protect the infant from acquiring the infection.

Other High Risk Groups

Many of the AIDS victims first identified were Haitian immigrants to Miami and New York City.[6,14,15] After the recognition of the syndrome in men and women from Haiti, it was soon appreciated that this was a problem of epidemic proportions in Haiti that had simply gone unreported.[15,20] Cases of invasive Kaposi's sarcoma, a disorder that was extremely rare before the appearance of AIDS, were appearing with increasing frequency in Port-au-Prince, Haiti, as early as 1980.[15] Homosexuality, drug abuse, and transfusions of infected blood clearly played no role in the increased incidence of AIDS in these immigrants.[6,14] The disease was assumed to have spread through heterosexual activity.

CASE HISTORY TWO

A previously healthy, 27-year-old Haitian woman was brought to the emergency room by her family after the abrupt onset of obtundation and hemiplegia. She had worked regularly until 2 weeks before this obtundation, at which time she began to complain of headaches. Five days before the emergency room visit, the patient developed difficulty speaking but retained language comprehension. Within a few days she was unable to walk and ate little.

The family reported that she had had a large lymph node in the supraclavicular region biopsied at another hospital 6 months earlier, but they had never learned the results of that biopsy. She had never received blood or blood products and did not abuse drugs or alcohol.

At the time of admission she had a fever of 105°F orally. She was responsive only to painful stimuli, to which she exhibited semi-purposeful movements of her right arm and leg. Her right pupil was slightly larger than her left and did not react to light. The left nasolabial fold was flattened and her eye movements were roving. Plantar responses were bilaterally upgoing. She had oral candidiasis.

Her white blood cell count was 5,400 cells/μL, and computed tomography of the brain revealed a right frontal lobe mass with surrounding edema and transfalcial herniation. While still in the emergency room, the patient rapidly deteriorated. She became unresponsive to deep pain and required respiratory support. She died within 2 days of admission.

An autopsy revealed cerebral toxoplasmosis in association with AIDS. There was a great deal of brain edema, and both the right uncus and the right cerebellar tonsil had herniated. One toxoplasma granuloma was visible grossly; a second, well-demarcated, yellow-tan, firm lesion with a distinct vascular rim was located in the right centrum semiovale. There were smaller areas of softening with discoloration scattered about the subcortical gray matter and in the cerebellum.

Microscopic examination of the largest granuloma revealed central necrosis with numerous toxoplasma cysts and nonencapsulated organisms. Surrounding the abscess, there was a thin rim of granulation tissue. Small arteries in the capsule exhibited severe vasculitis with mononuclear infiltrates involving the entire wall. Fibrin thrombi were evident in some of these vessels. There were numerous foci of microscopic hemorrhage and focal accumulations of neutrophils.

Damage to several components of the immune system were evident on pathologic examination. The patient had a necrotizing granulomatous lymphadenitis with parahilar lymph nodes prominent bilaterally. Lymphoid depletion and mild plasmacytosis were evident in the lymph nodes and thymus. Hassall's corpuscles were absent from the thymus.

How this woman acquired AIDS was never established. Although she was not a drug abuser, she had a rapidly progressive course with cerebral toxoplasmosis ultimately causing her death. The lethal problem was a right frontal granuloma that caused cerebral herniation. Masses caused by toxoplasmosis are common in patients with AIDS (Fig. 2-2).

Ironically, the incidence of seropositivity to HIV antibodies in Haitian immigrants was relatively low compared to that in other communities by 1984. Haitians in New York City had positive serums in less than 5 percent of the immigrants tested at the same time that seropositivity was found in over 87 percent of a group of intravenous drug abusers in the same city.[12] Identifying Haitians as a high risk group is no longer valid because the risk to the general pop-

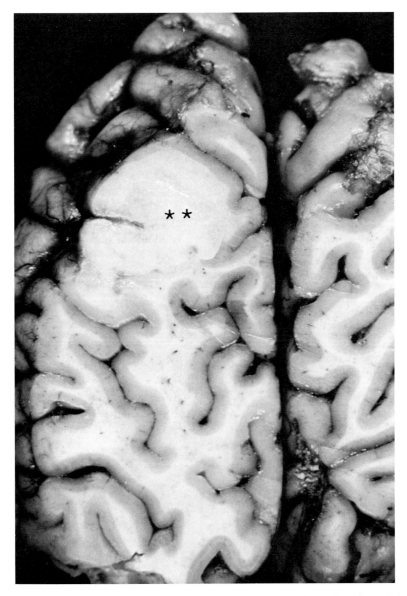

Fig. 2-2. Coronal section of the brain reveals a toxoplasma granuloma in the occipital lobe (asterisks).

ulation in the American cities where Haitians have settled is not very different from the risk in the non-Haitian population.

Immigrants and travelers from central Africa are still at high risk.[39] In equatorial Africa, AIDS is common in Zaire, Uganda, and at least 19 other nearby countries.[39,40]

In Uganda, it is known colloquially as "slim disease," a name alluding to the progressive weight loss seen in victims of the infection. The future of AIDS is suggested by the population statistics coming from central Africa: Men and women are equally affected and so are at equal risk of acquiring the infection.[39] HIV probably spreads primarily through heterosexual contact in Africa, but susceptibility studies on Africans and Europeans suggest that genetic factors may play a sizeable role in the dramatic spread of the virus in Africa.

Health care workers are regularly exposed to the virus, but well-documented incidents of infection through professional contact have been few.[16,23,35,41,42] Those workers developing AIDS have usually had contact with large volumes of contaminated blood, and most have had obvious breaks in the skin at the point of contact with the blood.[32,35] Individuals having more routine contact with contaminated materials, such as pathologists doing autopsies, gastroenterologists doing endoscopy, and technologists doing serum testing, have consistently tested negative.[42] It is possible that some of these individuals will eventually convert to seropositivity for HIV exposure, but current data do not suggest that the risk of acquiring AIDS in a hospital or laboratory setting is substantial even if the individuals working in these settings have direct contact with small amounts of contaminated material.[11,16,32,35,41,42]

In cities with high rates of AIDS cases, such as New York and San Francisco, physicians have adopted the attitude that anyone is at high risk. This may be excessively pessimistic, but it is appropriate in cities such as these where there has been more than 1 case of AIDS reported for every 1,000 members of the urban population. Although 67 percent of AIDS patients in the United States are white, 74 percent of the women with AIDS are black or Hispanic, and most are city-dwellers in their childbearing years.[22] This means that an increasing number of children born in urban centers like New York will acquire the virus before birth and die within months or years of birth as a consequence of that infection.

MECHANISMS FOR TRANSMISSION

Some of the mechanisms for the transmission of HIV from person to person have been discovered over the past few years, but many questions remain.[11,43] It is clear that body fluids other than blood and semen have viable virus: HIV has been isolated from saliva and tears.[35,41,44–48] That the virus can be transmitted by body fluids other than blood or semen is unlikely.[11,32,49] It is likely that cell-to-cell contact, rather than free viral attack on cells, is a major route, if not indeed *the* major route, for transmission of the infection.[43] This would explain why casual contact with infected individuals has not played a role in the spread of disease. The introduction of an infected individual's virus-laden cells directly into an uninfected individual's gastrointestinal tract, genitourinary tract, or bloodstream is the major route for transfer of the virus. There is substantial evidence that insects do not transmit the disease.[32,50]

Homosexual Transmission

Because AIDS appeared to require the introduction of infected material into the bloodstream, homosexual men acquiring the infection were assumed to have had rectal or anal tears. These lesions would allow the virus carried by semen to reach the vascular system during anal intercourse.[51] The virus is present in semen, both in the few white blood cells that are transported along with the spermatozoa and free in the seminal fluids.[47,52] The increased rate of AIDS transmission among individuals with venereal diseases may be both from the increased load of virus-laden lymphocytes in the sperm of men with venereal diseases and from the deterioration of skin and mucous membrane barriers to the virus when they are inflamed by bacterial or viral infections.

Breaks in the skin or rectal mucosa may provide a route for the transmission of the virus, but the spread of the disease in homosexual men has been much more rapid than a mechanism requiring trauma would suggest. What has been found is that homosexual male spread of the disease occurs primarily through anal intercourse, and the virus gains access to the victim's body through rectal mucosa cells. Whether this is done by release of the virus from infected cells which contact mucosal cells, by interactions between macrophages in the rectum of the anal-receptive partner and lymphocytes in the infected semen, or by invasion of rectal mucosal cells by free virions is unknown. The virus or infected lymphocyte might attach to receptors on the rectal mucosa that are similar or identical to the CD4 receptors on T lymphocytes.[33] Whether the virus can be acquired from an infected person by the anal-intrusive partner if that man has no lesions on the penis or in the urethra is unclear.

Heterosexual Transmission

Both men and women may contract AIDS through heterosexual activities. How HIV gains access to the bloodstream in heterosexual encounters is still unsettled, but that women can contract the virus through vaginal intercourse is indisputable. Indeed, women can develop AIDS even if their sexual partners have the human immunodeficiency virus but do not demonstrate any signs of the acquired immune deficiency syndrome. It is sufficient that a man has the virus to transmit it.[33]

Women contract AIDS four times as frequently through heterosexual activity as do men.[35] Why men face less risk of acquiring the disease through heterosexual activity is unknown. Women are believed to be capable of transmitting the virus to men during sexual intercourse, but the infectivity of the virus by way of vaginal secretions or discharges is apparently less than that by way of infected semen. Presumably the mucosal lining of the vagina and uterus are more easily invaded by the virus or virus infected cells than is the epidermis or urethral mucosa of the penis. For whatever reason, the spread of AIDS to strictly heterosexual men who do not abuse drugs and do not have hemophilia has been limited to relatively few cases.

The probability that a woman will be infected if her sexual partner carries the virus is high.[33] At least 23 percent of the women who have regular sexual activity with an infected man acquire the virus.[33] If the sexual partner acquired the infection through drug abuse, the probability that his female sexual partner will acquire the virus is greater than 40 percent.[33] The heterosexual partners of hemophiliacs have developed seropositivity for HIV antibodies in only 15 percent to 18 percent of cases after regular sexual activity with seropositive hemophiliacs.[25] The more sexual contact the woman has with the infected partner, the more likely she is to acquire the virus. Contact with only one man does not decrease the risk of infection if that man carries HIV.[33] Sexual activity with any individual who has an established HIV infection does not assure acquisition of the virus, but it certainly does pose a substantial risk to the uninfected sexual partner.

Promiscuity has not played a substantial role in the acquisition of AIDS by women. If none of a woman's sexual partners is a bisexual, an intravenous drug abuser, or a blood product recipient, her risk of acquiring the disease is not substantially increased by sexual activity with one or a dozen partners a week.[16,22] The limited risk posed by promiscuous behavior in groups that conscientiously avoid contact with drug abusing individuals and other members of high risk groups is ascribable to the still limited spread of the virus in the general population. Obviously, as more heterosexual individuals acquire the disease, the risk of acquiring the infection with each sexual encounter will increase.

If a woman has anal intercourse with an infected man, the virus will attach to the woman's rectal mucosa and subsequently invade macrophages and lymphocytes as in homosexual male encounters. This may partly explain the extensive heterosexual spread of AIDS in Africa. Female circumcision, a religious practice in which the clitoris is partly or completely amputated, is still widely practiced in several central African countries.[53] Some groups perform infibulation, in which the resection is so extensive that part of the vulva is resected and the resulting wound must be sewn together.[53] This practice narrows the vaginal entrance considerably and often makes vaginal intercourse painful. To avoid the pain for both partners, many heterosexual couples resort to anal intercourse.

Anal intercourse is also a common mode of birth control in areas lacking more conventional contraceptive strategies. American women who regularly engage in anal intercourse are twice as likely to acquire the infection from an infected sexual partner as are women who engage in strictly vaginal intercourse or fellatio.[33] These observations suggest that the virus is spread in many heterosexual couples by the same mechanisms it is spread in homosexual partners.

Concurrent venereal disease appears to increase the risk of heterosexual transmission of the AIDS virus.[22] Women with syphilis, gonorrhea, and other sexually transmitted diseases are at greater risk of acquiring the infection from an infected man than are women free of these other diseases. Genital ulcers in particular, whether they be from syphilis, herpes, or other infections, increase the probability that the exposed woman will acquire the infection.[22]

Intravenous Transmission

Although intravenous drug abusers were among the first groups recognized to be at risk for AIDS, safeguards against intravenous transmission of the virus are still inadequate. Drug abusers transmit the disease among themselves by sharing nonsterile hypodermic needles. HIV is a relatively unstable virus when left exposed to the elements, and so spread of the virus among drug abusers is probably accomplished by way of injection of infected cells.

Infected blood left in the hypodermic needle by an addict carrying HIV is introduced directly into the bloodstream of the uninfected addict who subsequently uses the needle. A small volume of blood appears to be sufficient to spread the infection, but repeated exposure to the virus may play a greater role in this method of spread than the risk entailed in individual exposures.[32] If the risk of acquiring the virus is only 1 in 100 each time an addict uses a contaminated needle, the addict will probably acquire the disease within a few months if most of the syringes available to him or her are contaminated.

Blood product recipients are at very low risk of being exposed to the virus because of intensive screening in blood banks in the United States and Europe, but hemophiliacs and other regular recipients of pooled blood products face a greater risk of acquiring the infection.[54] How much blood or blood product must be transfused to induce disease is unknown.[32] That the donor need not be symptomatic for HIV infection to transmit AIDS is well established. Indeed, blood from an HIV carrier may produce AIDS even if the donor does not develop AIDS until 2 years after donating the blood.[32] Once a donor's blood produces infection in a recipient, any future blood products acquired from that donor will transmit HIV infection.[32] This means that once an HIV infected individual has enough virus or enough competent virus in his or her blood to transmit the virus to a recipient, that donor will be permanently infectious.

The development of tests to check for antibodies to HIV has reduced the spread of the disease through transfusion, but there are still units of blood collected from individuals with viable HIV that test negative for antibodies to the virus with the techniques widely used. HIV infected blood is capable of transmitting AIDS even if antibodies to HIV are undetectable.[24] This means that further evaluation of blood and treatment of blood products before their use is necessary. This has been instituted in most industrialized countries.[25] Consequently, the risk of acquisition of HIV from appropriately handled blood in the United States is now less than 1 in 100,000 and is probably about 1 in 1,000,000.[32] This is important to children with newly recognized hemophilia and to individuals requiring blood transfusions, but it is irrelevant to the blood product recipients who acquired HIV between 1979 and 1987.

Intrauterine Transmission

Precisely how the AIDS virus crosses the placenta and infects the fetus is unknown. That it occurs is indisputable.[11,55] Transmission across the placenta is considered probable if the infant's mother is HIV positive and the child develops AIDS during the first 3 months of life.[56] The diagnosis of prenatally acquired AIDS is also accepted in premature infants if the HIV genome appears in thymic cells.[56]

No child has yet been described who acquired the infection before its mother. This means that HIV carried along with the sperm does not selectively infect the fertilized egg. Children who develop the infection more than 3 months after birth may have acquired the virus by transmission across the placenta or through contact with

maternal blood or secretion, such as breast milk.[38] Without a test that will establish the time of infection, children born to women with the virus are presumed to acquire the virus while in utero even if symptoms of disease do not appear until several years after birth. Early detection of antibodies in the newborn has limited usefulness in establishing the presence of HIV in the child since these antibodies may be transmitted from the infected mother.

Free virus is not likely to be circulating in maternal blood if the woman is healthy enough to sustain a pregnancy, and so transmission across the placenta is probably by way of infected maternal cells. Monocytes or monocytes that have differentiated into macrophages may migrate into the placenta and defeat the physiologic barriers that this interface provides. Even if the macrophages are rapidly destroyed as they breach the placenta, the virus they carry could readily invade fetal monocytes and lymphocytes.

Other Routes of Spread

One of the growing fears about the transmission of AIDS is that the virus might be transmissible by an insect vector, such as mosquitoes or ticks. There has been no evidence that this is possible, although HIV has been recovered from mosquitoes that have ingested heavily contaminated blood meals prepared under laboratory conditions.[50] The virus in these mosquitoes is still viable 48 hours after ingestion, but there is no evidence that the virus can multiply in the mosquito or enter the insect's saliva, as occurs with viruses that are transmitted by mosquitoes.[50] The amount of blood left in the insect's mouthparts, even immediately after a blood meal, is generally not considered sufficient to be infectious.[50] In diseases transmitted by mosquitoes, the virus is usually present at high concentrations in the anticoagulant saliva that is actively injected into the victim at the moment the proboscis of the insect punctures the skin.

Acquisition of the virus during casual contact with an AIDS victim has generally been discounted, but contact with heavily infected blood may allow transmission of the disease.[11,35] Presumably the virus cannot gain access to the bloodstream through intact epidermis, but small cuts and punctures of the skin are common enough to place anyone soiled with contaminated blood at risk of acquiring the infection. A few health care workers who did get large volumes of blood on their skin have developed AIDS.[35] As of June, 1987, the Centers for Disease Control in the United States had identified nine health care workers who had acquired HIV but who had no risk factors other than that they were exposed to patients or patient materials with AIDS virus.[16] This constitutes much too small a group of individuals to suggest that health care workers are in a high risk category.

GEOGRAPHIC DISTRIBUTION

The AIDS virus seems to have arisen or at least flourished for some time on the western shore of Lake Victoria in central Africa. A retrovirus similar to HIV-1 and HIV-2 was isolated from wild African Green monkeys, and this monkey virus was subsequently found in people along trade routes from central Africa to West Africa. In female prostitutes in Senegal, West Africa, the monkey virus is still evident.[57] After being transmitted to humans, the monkey retrovirus may have mutated to the lethal HIV-2.[58] Presumably HIV-2 subsequently mutated to the more widespread HIV-1.[59]

That these viruses are especially susceptible to mutation is evident from the variety of strains of HIV-1 isolated in Europe, Africa, and the United States.[58] Strains of the human immunodeficiency virus appearing in Africa are more like the African Green monkey retrovirus than are HIV strains from the United States.[57] How the African Green monkey retrovirus or a related virus that gave rise to HIV-2 was transmitted to humans is unknown.

How long ago the virus first appeared in Africa is open to speculation, but studies on frozen serum samples suggest that the virus was in Uganda, Tanzania, Kenya, and the Ivory Coast as long ago as 1970.[57,60,61] Some investigators believe that they have found evidence of the virus in samples from Kinshasa dating back to 1959.[57] Evaluation of these frozen specimens is difficult because of the high level of false-positive results in specimens from areas with high levels of malaria and other tropical diseases.[62] That the virus was in Africans before 1974 is debatable, but that it was prevalent before 1981 is indisputable.[61] Sporadic cases occurring before 1970 in widely scattered locations, including the United States, indicate that this virus has existed for more than one decade and perhaps much longer. It is quite possible that it has been widespread for centuries and only rarely mutated to the lethal form that is now causing the AIDS epidemic.

Over the past decade, HIV has been transmitted along the central African highway, which carries commerce to both the east and west of Lake Victoria. Prostitutes traveling along this highway with work crews and truckers have probably been the principal carriers of the virus from one major city to the next. In the 1960s, many Haitian teachers in search of employment went to Zaire because passports to that country were readily available to educated Haitians. Zaire needed French-speaking teachers in many areas to fill positions formerly held by the French who were no longer active in Zaire because of their declining interest in previously French-controlled African colonies. The French-speaking Haitians were paid less than the French, but salaries available in Zaire allowed for a much higher standard of living than that available to unemployed teachers in Haiti. It is likely that these Haitians brought the virus back to Haiti from Africa when they returned home.

Transmission of the virus from Haiti to the United States was also prompted by poverty. Haiti was a favorite vacation spot for many homosexual men. The cost of food, shelter, and sexual partners was very low. Male prostitutes transmitted the disease to the vacationing men. When the disease was first recognized in major urban centers of the United States, such as New York, epidemiologic studies quickly identified homosexual men and recently arriving Haitians as two groups with inordinately high rates of infection with the AIDS virus.

Political responses to evidence of the epidemic only helped to spread it. In central Africa, evidence of widespread disease was denied by political leaders who were concerned about the economic effects of such news.[39] Until 1986, there were no official reports of any cases of AIDS in central Africa, despite medical evidence of an epidemic.[39] A study performed by the Hôpital Claude Bernard in Paris found that the prevalence of antibodies to HIV in serum from prostitutes in Kenya rose from 7 percent in 1980 to 51 percent in 1984.[39] Men in Kenya who sought medical attention for other sexually transmitted diseases had an increase in positive antibody tests from 1 percent in 1980 to 13 percent in 1984.[39] In Rwanda, more than 10 percent of blood donations collected throughout the country contained antibodies to the AIDS virus, but more than 17 percent of those coming from urban areas were positive in 1985.[39]

In Haiti, the political leadership did not collect statistics on the spreading infection, and economic considerations again helped to suppress the mounting evidence of a rapidly spreading epidemic. In the United States, recognition of the disease and concern about its spread developed soon after the first patients died with the disease, but

identification of homosexual men and Haitian immigrants as the carriers of the disease resulted in counterproductive reactions by representatives of both groups and by politicians sensitive to the indignation of both groups. Efforts to identify carriers of the virus were frustrated by concern for the privacy of individuals and fear that the singling out of specific groups would produce divisive sanctions against those groups. Shortsighted efforts to frustrate the identification of individuals carrying the virus provided an opportunity for the virus to spread to initially unaffected members of the population.

Individuals testing positive for the virus were not necessarily told that they could transmit the infection, and their sexual partners, both homosexual and heterosexual, became infected. Routine quarantine measures were not enforced. Standard containment procedures were not introduced. Testing of the population through previously accepted measures for detecting sexually transmitted diseases, such as premarital and hospital admission testing, was not adopted. As if to satisfy those who were outraged by the identification of a small segment of the population carrying the virus, the infection spread to all sectors of the population.

Over 100 countries now report cases of AIDS.[16] International projections suggest that 3 million people will develop AIDS by 1992, and there is no region that has substantially resisted encroachment by the AIDS virus.[16] The disease is a global problem and will require a global strategy.

Knowledge of where the virus originated is only useful in helping to identify related viruses that may simplify the development of a vaccine. HIV has spread to cities all over the world and can no longer be sequestered without Draconian measures that would isolate millions of affected individuals. The true prevalence of the disease in most countries is still unknown because of widespread resistance to testing for HIV antibodies.

REFERENCES

1. Hooper DC, Pruitt AA, Rubin RH: Central nervous system infections in the chronically immunosuppressed. Medicine (Baltimore) 61:166, 1982
2. Miller JR, Barrett RE, Britton CG, et al: Progressive multifocal leukoencephalopathy in a male homosexual with T-cell immune deficiency. N Engl J Med 307:1436, 1982
3. Centers for Disease Control Task Force on Kaposi's Sarcoma and Opportunistic Infections: Epidemiologic aspects of the current outbreak of Kaposi's sarcoma and opportunistic infections. N Engl J Med 306:248, 1982
4. Drew WL, Conant MA, Miner RC, et al: Cytomegalovirus and Kaposi's sarcoma in young homosexual men. Lancet 2:125, 1982
5. Gopinathan G, Laubenstein LJ, Mondale B, Krigel RL: Central nervous system manifestations of the acquired immunodeficiency (AID) syndrome in homosexual men. Neurology 33:suppl 2, 105, 1983
6. Moskowitz LB, Kory P, Chan JC, et al: Unusual causes of death in Haitians residing in Miami: high prevalence of opportunistic infections. JAMA 250:1187, 1983
7. Pitchenik AE, Fischl MA, Walls KW: Evaluation of cerebral mass lesions in acquired immunodeficiency syndrome. N Engl J Med 308:1099, 1983
8. Harris C, Small CB, Klein RS, et al: Immunodeficiency among female sexual partners of males with acquired immunodeficiency syndrome. N Engl J Med 308:1181, 1983
9. Barré-Sinoussi F, Chermann J-C, Rey F, et al: Isolation of a T-lymphotropic retrovirus from a patient at risk for acquired immune deficiency syndrome (AIDS). Science 220:868, 1983
10. Gallo RC, Salahuddin SZ, Popovic M, et al: Frequent detection and isolation of cytopathic retroviruses (HTLV-III) from patients with AIDS and at risk for AIDS. Science 224:500, 1984
11. Sande M: Transmission of AIDS: the case against contagion. N Engl J Med 341:380, 1986
12. Landesman SH, Ginzburg HM, Weiss SH: The AIDS epidemic. N Engl J Med 312:521, 1985
13. Marx JL: Probing the AIDS virus and its relatives. Science 236:1523, 1987
14. Vieira J, Frank E, Spira TJ, Landesman SH: Acquired immune deficiency in Haitians. N Engl J Med 308:125, 1983
15. Pitchenik AE, Fischl MA, Dickinson GM, et al: Opportunistic infections and Kaposi's sarcoma among Haitians: evidence of a new acquired immunodeficiency state. Ann Intern Med 98:277, 1983
16. Barnes DM: AIDS: statistics but few answers. Science 237:1423, 1987
17. Booth W: Experts fault leadership on AIDS. Science 237:838, 1987
18. Wykoff R: Female-to-male transmission of AIDS agent. Lancet 2:1017, 1985
19. Hardy AM, Allen JR, Morgan WM, et al: The incidence rate of acquired immunodeficiency syndrome in selected populations. JAMA 253:215, 1985
20. Levy RM, Bredesen DE, Rosenblum ML: Neurologic manifestations of the acquired immunodeficiency syndrome (AIDS): experience at the University of California at San Francisco and review of the literature. J Neurosurg 62:475, 1985
21. Polk BF, Fox R, Brookmeyer R, et al: Predictors of the acquired immunodeficiency syndrome developing in a cohort of seropositive homosexual men. N Engl J Med 316:61, 1987
22. Edwards DD: Heterosexuals and AIDS: mixed messages. Science News 132:60, 1987
23. Essex M, McLane MF, Lee TH, et al: Antibodies to human T-cell leukemia virus membrane antigens (HTLV-MA) in hemophiliacs. Science 221:1061, 1983
24. Davis KC, Horsburgh CR, Jr, Hasiba U, et al: Acquired immunodeficiency syndrome in a patient with hemophilia. Ann Intern Med 98:284, 1983
25. Hilgartner MW: AIDS and hemophilia. N Engl J Med 317:1153, 1987
26. Desforges J: AIDS and preventive treatment in hemophilia. N Engl J Med 308:94, 1983
27. AIDS Weekly Surveillance Report: United States AIDS Program, Atlanta: Public Health Service, Centers for Infectious Diseases, Centers for Disease control, February 2, 1987

28. Evatt B, Gomperts E, McDougal J, et al: Coincidental appearance of LAV/HTLV-III antibodies in hemophiliacs and the onset of the AIDS epidemic. N Engl J Med 312:483, 1985
29. Curran J: The epidemiology and prevention of acquired immunodeficiency syndrome. Ann Intern Med 103:657, 1985
30. CDC: Human immunodeficiency virus infection in transfusion recipients and their family members. MMWR 36:137–140, 1987
31. Shannon KM, Amman AJ: Acquired immune deficiency syndrome in childhood. J Pediatr 106:332, 1985
32. Friedland GH, Klein RS: Transmission of human immunodeficiency virus. N Engl J Med 317:1125, 1987
33. Edwards DD: High-risk sex studied in women, men. Science News 132:116, 1987
34. Fischl MA, Dickson GM, Scott GM, et al: Evaluation of heterosexual partners, children, and household contacts of adults with AIDS. JAMA 257:640, 1987
35. FDA: Special AIDS issue. FDA Drug Bull 17:14–24, 1987
36. Guinan ME, Hardy A: Epidemiology of AIDS in women in the United States: 1981 through 1986. JAMA 257:2039, 1987
37. Epstein LG, Sharer LR, Oleske JM, et al: Neurologic manifestations of human immunodeficiency virus infection in children. Pediatrics 78:678, 1986
38. Ziegler JB, Cooper DA, Johnson RO, et al: Postnatal transmission of AIDS-associated retrovirus from mother to infant. Lancet 1:896, 1985
39. Normal C: Politics and science clash on African AIDS. Science 230:1140, 1985
40. Mann J, Quinn TC, Piot P, et al: Condom use and HIV infection among prostitutes in Zaire. N Engl J Med 316:345, 1987
41. CDC: Update: human immunodeficiency virus infections in health-care workers exposed to blood of infected patients. MMWR 36:285, 1987
42. Hirsch MS, Wormser GP, Schooley RT, et al: Risk of nosocomial infection with human T-cell lymphotropic virus III (HTLV-III). N Engl J Med 312:1, 1985
43. Marx JL: The AIDS virus—well known but a mystery. Science 236:390, 1987
44. CDC: Recommendations for preventing possible transmission of HTLV-III/LAV from tears. MMWR 34:533, 1985
45. CDC: Recommendations for preventing transmission of infection with human T-lymphotropic virus type III/lymphadenopathy-associated virus during invasive procedures. MMWR 35:221, 1986
46. Groopman JE, Salahuddin SZ, Sarngadharan MG, et al: HTLV-III in saliva of people with AIDS-related complex and healthy homosexual men at risk for AIDS. Science 226:447, 1984
47. Zagury D, Bernard J, Leibowitch J, et al: HTLV-III in cells cultured from semen of two patients with AIDS. Science 226:449, 1984
48. Fujikawa LS, Salahuddin SZ, Palestine AG, et al: Isolation of human T-lymphotropic virus type III from the tears of a patient with the acquired immunodeficiency syndrome. Lancet 2:529, 1985
49. Curran JW, Morgan WM, Hardy AM, et al: The epidemiology of AIDS: current status and future prospects. Science 229:1352, 1985
50. Booth W: AIDS and insects. Science 237:355, 1987
51. Jaffe HW, Choi K, Thomas PA, et al: National case-control study of Kaposi's sarcoma and pneumocystic carinii pneumonia in homosexual men: Part 1. Epidemiologic results. Ann Intern Med 99:145, 1983
52. Ho DD, Schooley RT, Rota TR, et al: HTLV-III in the semen and blood of a healthy homosexual man. Science 226:451, 1984
53. Linke U: AIDS in Africa. Science 230:203, 1986
54. Allain J-P, Laurian Y, Paul DA, et al: Long-term evaluation of HIV antigen and antibodies to p24 and gp41 in patients with hemophilia. N Engl J Med 317:1114, 1987
55. Rogers MF: AIDS in children: a review of the clinical, epidemiologic and public health aspects. Pediatr Infect Dis 4:230, 1985
56. Case 9-1986: A 40-month-old girl with the acquired immunodeficiency syndrome and spinal-cord compression. N Engl J Med 314:629, 1986
57. Normal C: Africa and the origin of AIDS. Science 230:1141, 1985
58. Kanki PJ, M'Boup S, Ricard D, et al:

Human T-lymphotropic virus type 4 and the human immunodeficiency virus in West Africa. Science 236:827, 1987

59. Gnann JW, McCormick JB, Mitchell S, et al: Synthetic peptide immunoassay distinguishes HIV type 1 and HIV type 2 infections. Science 237:1346, 1987

60. Brun-Vezinet F, Rouzioux C, Montagnier L, et al: Prevalence of antibodies to lymph-adenopathy-associated retrovirus in African patients with AIDS. Science 226:453, 1984

61. Quinn TC, Mann JM, Curran JW, Piot P: AIDS in Africa: an epidemiologic paradigm. Science 234:955, 1986

62. Sher R, Antunes S, Reid R, Falcke H: Seroepidemiology of human immunodeficiency virus in Africa from 1970 to 1974. N Engl J Med 317:450, 1987

3

Neurologic Involvement

The nervous system is routinely an early and obvious site of disease in acquired immune deficiency syndrome (AIDS).[1-4] In addition to the opportunistic infections that the defect in cell-mediated immunity allows, there is neurologic damage directly attributable to the AIDS virus.[5-9] The human immunodeficiency virus (HIV) directly attacks cells in the nervous system, although it does not cause morphologic injury to neurons.[10,11] It causes disabling, but not necessarily irreversible, damage to the brain and spinal cord.[12-14] The most common manifestation of this viral injury is a progressive dementia associated with a subacute encephalitis or encephalopathy. Spinal cord, cranial nerve, and peripheral nerve damage also occur but are much less likely to dominate the clinical picture in the patient with AIDS than is the AIDS-related encephalopathy.[15,16]

What fraction of the AIDS population develops nervous system damage from the retrovirus is unknown, but HIV probably invades the nervous system in the majority of AIDS cases.[17,18] Although there is some evidence that HTLV-I causes spinal cord damage in susceptible individuals, HIV is the only retrovirus that has unequivocally been demonstrated to attack the human nervous system. As already discussed in Chapter 1, HIV is a member of the lentiviral subfamily of retroviruses. Past experience with lentiviral diseases in a variety of other animals suggests what types of problems may be direct effects of the lentivirus on the nervous system.[19,20] As is true for visna, the retroviral cousin of HIV that attacks sheep, the central nervous system is more often and more directly impaired by the AIDS virus than is the peripheral nervous system.[15,19] Vacuolar changes in myelin and areas of demyelination are more obvious than inflammation or neuronal loss in most lentiviral diseases.

Patients with HIV infection do not necessarily have immune system failure before nervous system signs and neuropathologic changes are induced by the virus. This means that even if strategies are developed to protect the immune system from HIV, the nervous system will not necessarily be protected from the retrovirus. Patients with immune systems adequately intact to stave off opportunistic infections in the nervous system and elsewhere may still develop subacute encephalitis, progressive myelopathy, aseptic meningitis, and peripheral neuropathy caused by HIV.[15]

EARLY SIGNS OF AIDS

Although signs of nervous system disease may appear early in the course of AIDS, the patient's initial complaints usually are not neurologic. These complaints often include generalized malaise, shortness of

Table 3-1. Systemic Problems in Patients with CNS AIDS

Systemic Disease	Prevalence (%)
Pneumocystis carinii pneumonia	67
Cytomegalovirus infection	67
Oropharyngeal candidiasis	47
Kaposi's sarcoma	33
Perianal *Herpes simplex*	30
Toxoplasma gondii infection	17
Viral hepatitis	17
Mycobacterium avium intracellulare	10
Cryptococcus neoformans	7
Varicella zoster	3

Based on data from de la Monte et al.[42]

breath, and easy fatigability.[15,21] These signs and symptoms suggest nonneurologic infection and are usually manifestations of a *Pneumocystis carinii* pneumonia[1] (Table 3-1). Early physical signs of AIDS also include generalized lymphadenopathy, refractory fungal infections, recurrent diarrhea, and intractable weight loss associated with lymphopenia.[21,22] Some patients have no strictly neurologic signs or symptoms evident when they initially become symptomatic for AIDS, but the majority develop obvious neurologic disease before they die.[1] The mean interval from nonneurologic presentation of AIDS to neurologic illness in those who eventually become symptomatic is only 5 months.[1]

In many cases of AIDS, the first problems suggest a central or peripheral nervous system disturbance. If symptoms referable to the nervous system antedate complaints of shortness of breath and generalized malaise, they are often psychiatric and nonspecific.[23,24] Depression is an especially common premonitory complaint, and personality changes, social withdrawal, lethargy, and reduced libido are also evident.[21] Psychomotor retardation often accompanies these early signs.[24]

As many as 39 percent of patients with AIDS have neurologic signs or symptoms at the time of their initial examination, and at least 63 percent develop neurologic problems before they die.[1,22] In some patients,

neurologic signs and symptoms are the only clinical manifestations of HIV infection.[25] At autopsy, 80 percent to 90 percent of patients with AIDS have neuropathologic abnormalities, even if they had no neurologic disturbances evident before death.[26,27] Neurologic symptoms in the AIDS victim range from mild confusion and poor coordination to profound dementia and disabling ataxia.[25,28]

If dementia develops early in the disease, it is likely to go unrecognized unless it is severe. Lapses of memory, mildly disturbed speech, and problems with orientation are usually dismissed by the medically unsophisticated as unimportant.[23] Over weeks to months, infected patients may develop progressive dementia, psychomotor retardation, bladder and bowel incontinence, disorientation, and hallucinations.[25] These neurologic signs are not specific for any one type of neurologic complication of AIDS but may occur with subacute encephalitis, opportunistic infections, cerebral neoplasms, or even as remote signs of systemic infection.

The most common cause of neurologic signs and symptoms in patients with AIDS is central nervous system infection[1] Table 3-2), which may be an encephalitis or a meningitis caused by an opportunistic infection. Many patients exhibit multiple neurologic disorders, the most common problem associated with multiple neurologic problems in patients with AIDS being retinitis, pre-

Table 3-2. CNS Disease with AIDS

Disease	Prevalence (%)
HIV subacute encephalitis	90
HIV vacuolar myelopathy	11–22
HIV aseptic meningitis	5–10
Toxoplasmosis	17
Cryptococcosis	7
Cytomegalovirus infection	7
Lymphoma	7
Mycobacterial infection	3
Progressive multifocal leukoencephalopathy	3

Based on data from de la Monte et al.[42] and Gabuzda DH et al.[15]

sumably from cytomegalovirus or toxoplasmosis in the majority of cases.[1] Neuropathies, radiculopathies, myopathies, and cerebrovascular disease all occur in patients with AIDS; but none is nearly so common as the meningoencephalitides that develop with this syndrome.[1]

Any patient with AIDS believed to have signs of central nervous system disease (CNS) must be rigorously investigated. Noninvasive tests are usually inadequate to determine the precise character of the CNS disease. Most patients require cerebrospinal fluid analysis; some require brain biopsies. Every investigation must be pursued rapidly and aggressively because of the high probability of lethal complications in patients with central nervous system disease.

NEUROLOGIC SIGNS OF HIV INFECTION

That HIV finds its way into a variety of tissues in the central and peripheral nervous system is well established.[9,29,30] The human immunodeficiency virus has been isolated from many nervous system components, including the cerebrospinal fluid, brain, spinal cord, cornea, and peripheral nerves, of affected individuals.[8,9,11,16,20,31] HIV causes an encephalitis and a myelitis as a direct consequence of central nervous system spread of the virus, but the symptoms associated with this may be quite subtle until the encephalomyelitis is advanced.[24,32] A demyelinating peripheral neuropathy also develops, probably as a direct effect of HIV infection. Whether the unexplained myositis observed in some patients with AIDS is a direct effect of HIV or of another infectious agent is still controversial.[33]

Because the types of neurologic problems directly attributable to HIV have been recognized for relatively few years, the terminology used to identify these problems is somewhat inconsistent. The subacute encephalomyelitis caused by HIV has been referred to as AIDS-related encephalopathy, AIDS dementia complex, subacute encephalitis, and HIV encephalopathy. Subacute encephalomyelitis is the most accurate name for this inflammatory retroviral disease of the brain and spinal cord, but it has not been widely adopted.

Human immunodeficiency virus apparently disturbs central nervous system function in several ways. It may harm cells in the nervous system by infecting them or by interfering with the binding of substances to receptors on the surface of the cells.[9,34,35] By whatever means this retrovirus causes its effects on the nervous system, its attack on nervous tissue does not exclude other organisms from also infecting the nervous system. Much of the neurologic disease apparent in patients with AIDS is from opportunistic infections, rather than from HIV itself, but even patients with toxoplasmosis, cryptococcosis, or cytomegalovirus infections may have pathologic evidence of concurrent damage to nervous system tissues by HIV.

Much of the pathophysiology of HIV infection in the nervous system is unresolved. How and when the virus gets into the nervous system after it is acquired by the patient is unknown. Many investigators believe that HIV enters the nervous system in infected monocytes or macrophages.[11,16] Once in the central nervous system, the virus may invade nervous system tissue, perhaps because components of the immune system and of the nervous system have similar receptors.[34] The chain of events occurring in the brain once HIV has established itself there is obviously complex.[9] The virus does not simply attack cell after cell, destroying vital elements of the nervous system as it spreads. In fact, there appears to be considerable variability in precisely what effect the virus will have on the host nervous tissues. The strains of HIV surviving in the central nervous system apparently vary, with some exhibiting neu-

Table 3-3. The Diagnosis of HIV Encephalopathy

Epidemiology	Usually a member of high risk group
Clinical presentation	Dementia, bradykinesia, tremor, ataxia, paraparesis, social withdrawal, psychosis
Neurodiagnostic findings	Brain atrophy and white matter changes on CT or MRI Multinucleated giant cells, microglial nodules, and demyelination on brain biopsy
Systemic findings	AIDS, pre-AIDS, or systemically asymptomatic
Immunologic findings	Helper-inducer lymphocyte (CD4) count less than 400/µL; CD4/CD8 ratio reversed
Serologic findings	HIV antibodies by ELISA or other method
Cultures	HIV in blood, cerebrospinal fluid, or brain tissue

ropathic potentials and others not exhibiting any destructive capabilities.[11,36]

Subacute Encephalitis

The most common site for neurologic problems with AIDS is the central nervous system, and the most common cause of disturbed nervous system function in AIDS is subacute encephalitis secondary to human immunodeficiency virus (HIV) infection[24,31] (see Table 3-2). Because dementia is so prominent a feature of this encephalitis, many investigators have called it the AIDS dementia complex.[9,37–40] Dementia is recognizable as a distinct problem in at least two-thirds of individuals with AIDS.[25,35] Its significance in patients with HIV infection prompted the Centers for Disease Control to include it in their definition of AIDS.[18]

This encephalitis may be the initial or sole clinical manifestation of HIV infection, but usually it is one of several problems affecting the patient[9,25] (Table 3-3). That it occurs independently of severe immunosuppression is well established, but that it occurs as a product of cell death after HIV infection is less evident.[25] This is a central nervous system disease that does not restrict itself to the brain but usually extends to the spinal cord, as well. Perhaps 90 percent of patients who die with AIDS and central nervous system disease have a subacute encephalitis or encephalomyelitis attributable to HIV.[32,41,42] An aseptic meningitis attributable to HIV may occur along with the subacute encephalitis or independently.[42]

CLINICAL FINDINGS

Early in the course of HIV subacute encephalitis the patient appears depressed and has a blunted affect.[21,23] Impaired memory, poor concentration, and social withdrawal are usually evident[21,25] (Table 3-4). Cognitive deterioration routinely evolves over the course of months.[37] In 80 percent of patients, profound dementia is evident within a year of the appearance of symptoms.[15,37] Patients occasionally have a more rapid deterioration in cognitive abilities, with dementia progressing over the course of days rather than months. This rapid course is usually associated with systemic problems, such as an evolving pulmonary infection with hypoxia, and may be a combination of the AIDS associated dementia and a metabolic encephalopathy.

Other neurologic problems, such as loss of balance, movement disorders, or paraparesis, routinely appear along with the evolving dementia.[37–39] Behavioral changes may be quite prominent; more than one-

Table 3-4. Signs and Symptoms of HIV Subacute Encephalitis

Early	Late
Forgetfulness	Psychomotor slowing
Loss of balance	Gait ataxia
Slight leg weakness	Paraparesis
Social withdrawal	Psychosis
Apathy	Frontal lobe release signs
Depression	Akinetic mutism
Tremor	Myoclonus
	Incontinence
	Spasticity
	Seizures

Table 3-5. Movement Disorders with HIV Infection

Segmental myoclonus
Supranuclear ophthalmoplegia
Parkinsonian tremor
Postural tremor
Chorea
Hemiballismus
Limb dystonia

third of the patients affected will exhibit apathy, social withdrawal, emotional lability, or other obvious behavioral disturbances.[37] Some patients become delusional and disoriented.[21] Cognitive deficits extend to involve speech. Eventually the patient becomes mute. Seizures may occur, and terminally the patient is usually comatose.[21]

Movement disorders develop early in the course of disease in some patients with AIDS encephalopathy (Table 3-5). In rare patients a movement disorder is the first clinical sign of HIV infection.[43] Tremors and myoclonus have been reported in several patients.[25,43,44] Rigidity in association with the tremors and segmental dystonia, such as torticollis, develop in some patients. Chorea and more complex movement disorders have occurred primarily in patients with AIDS complicated by cerebral toxoplasmosis or cerebral Whipple's disease.[43] All patients with HIV subacute encephalitis eventually develop motor signs, the most common being ataxia, paraparesis, and tremors.[25]

Those who are conscious late in the evolution of this subacute encephalopathy often have ataxia, hypertonia, incontinence, tremors, and limb weakness, as well as profound dementia.[37] Death in most demented patients results from aspiration pneumonia or a systemic opportunistic infection.[37] The mean survival time varies with the severity of the patient's immunosuppression. Patients with obvious signs of immunosuppression survive about 6 months; those with dementia as their primary problem, and little evidence of immunodeficiency, usually survive about 9 months.[25]

Case History One

A 31-year-old woman was admitted because of progressive deterioration of short-term memory, increasing lethargy, sleeplessness, and tremors. These signs had all become prominent over the 2 weeks before hospital admission. Six years before the current hospitalization, she had been admitted for management of an ectopic pregnancy. She received a blood transfusion at that time and subsequently had a long-term sexual relationship with an intravenous-drug-abusing boyfriend. Three years after the ectopic pregnancy, she developed viral pneumonia, which was not characterized but resolved, and chronic fatigue and pharyngitis, which did not resolve. One year before her final admission, she developed non-A, non-B hepatitis, which was considered a chronic active hepatitis on the basis of a liver biopsy.

Physical examination at the time of the final admission revealed enlarged cervical and axillary lymph nodes. In addition to short-term memory loss, her intellectual function was disturbed by paranoid delusions. She was tremulous, lethargic, and uncooperative and had athetoid movements of the limbs and myoclonic jerks.

Initial laboratory tests revealed abnormal liver function tests and elevated cerebrospinal fluid protein content (83 mg/dL). Subsequently the cerebrospinal fluid also contained an increased number of mononuclear cells (18/μL). Computed tomography of the brain revealed diffuse atrophy with mild ventricular dilation. Magnetic resonance imaging (MRI) suggested focal structural changes in the tip of the right temporal lobe, the posterior limb of the right internal capsule, and in the periventricular white matter bilaterally. None of these focal changes was associated with any mass effect or edema. The electroencephalogram showed diffuse slowing of the background activity.

Three weeks after admission she developed hallucinations, increasing lethargy, headache, and low-grade fever. Her serum ammonia level reached 80, but the cerebral lesions justified a brain biopsy. A right temporal lobe biopsy revealed small microglial nodules with multinucleated giant cells in the cerebral cortex and white matter. The histologic picture was that of AIDS-associated subacute encephalitis. Cerebral toxoplasmosis was incidentally identified.

After surgery, the patient developed a left hemiparesis, pneumonia, and progressive obtundation. She died shortly thereafter.

This patient developed cognitive problems and movement disorders early in the course of her disease, a disease acquired either from a blood transfusion or from a drug-abusing sexual partner. As is often true with HIV encephalitis, there was evidence of an opportunistic infection in the central nervous system. Ascertaining which signs and symptoms are attributable to HIV encephalitis and which are attributable to the opportunistic infections becomes more difficult as the patient becomes increasingly ill. The pathologic findings in this patient of multinucleated giant cells and microglial nodules scattered throughout the cerebrum are typical of HIV encephalopathy.

DIAGNOSTIC TESTS

Diagnostic tests short of brain biopsy are fairly unrevealing. The cerebrospinal fluid is often normal except for a mild elevation of cerebrospinal fluid protein content or a low-grade mononuclear pleocytosis.[15,22,37] The protein content usually does not exceed 200 mg/dL.[37] Oligoclonal IgG bands are detectable in some patients, but this is not helpful in establishing the diagnosis.[37] Identifying HIV or HIV antibodies in the cerebrospinal fluid of patients with AIDS is also not helpful in establishing the diagnosis of HIV subacute encephalitis because HIV antigens and antibodies routinely appear in the

CSF of patients with AIDS who have no evidence of progressive neuropathology.[45]

The electroencephalogram exhibits diffuse, but nonspecific, slowing.[15,22,25] Computed tomography and magnetic resonance imaging of the brain show mild cortical atrophy or no gross changes at all.[22,37] If there is cerebral cortical atrophy, there is usually an associated hydrocephalus ex vacuo.[25]

Of considerable importance in arriving at the diagnosis of HIV encephalopathy is the demonstration of reduced helper-inducer (T4) T lymphocyte counts in the peripheral blood or an inverted CD4/CD8 T lymphocyte ratio.[25] The patient need not have advanced immune deficiency, but hematologic parameters should be disturbed. HIV seropositivity is also useful. Patients with probable AIDS encephalopathy will require brain biopsy to determine that the brain injury is not from a specific opportunistic infection. Southern blot analysis and in situ hybridization will establish the presence of HIV nucleic acid in brain tissues.[25,46]

HISTOPATHOLOGY

In one-third of patients with AIDS and signs of neurologic disease, the neuropathologic changes in the central nervous system are remarkably minor[3,6,37] (Table 3-6). Glial changes may dominate all other path-

Table 3-6. Histopathologic Features of Subacute Encephalitis

Feature	Prevalence (%)
White matter gliosis	96
Fibrillary gliosis of gray matter	89
Focal necrosis	81
Microglial nodules	70
Atypical oligodendrocytes	63
Perivascular inflammation	52
Demyelination	44
Axonal spheroids	41
Multinucleated giant cells	33
Leptomeningeal inflammation	19
Vacuolar myelopathy	11

Based on data from de la Monte et al.[70] and Gabuzda et al.[71]

ologic findings. The inflammatory reactions mounted with HIV infection are much less prominent than those mounted in other subacute encephalitides. If inflammatory changes are evident, they are most likely to be found in the cortical white matter and deep gray matter structures, including the basal ganglia.[9,25]

The extent of inflammation and the severity of dementia in patients with HIV subacute encephalitis do not correlate with the length of time the patient has carried the diagnosis of AIDS.[42] In some patients this may be more a function of the changing definition of AIDS than of the length of time the patient has had HIV infection.[18] Patients who would have been considered AIDS risks in 1983 are now unequivocally diagnosed as AIDS patients.

Structural and Microscopic Changes

Grossly, little is evident with HIV subacute encephalitis other than some white matter pallor and diffuse cerebral atrophy.[25] More is evident on microscopic examination of the affected brain; but neither the structural nor the microscopic findings in HIV encephalitis explain the dementia that routinely develops. Microglial nodules are especially prominent in HIV subacute encephalitis[42] (Fig. 3-1). Microglial nodules are clusters of mononuclear cells, presumed to arise from macrophages and microglia, that occur in several different inflammatory diseases of the central nervous system.[16] In HIV encephalitis they develop around blood vessels in many different parts of the brain. Neuronal loss is not associated with

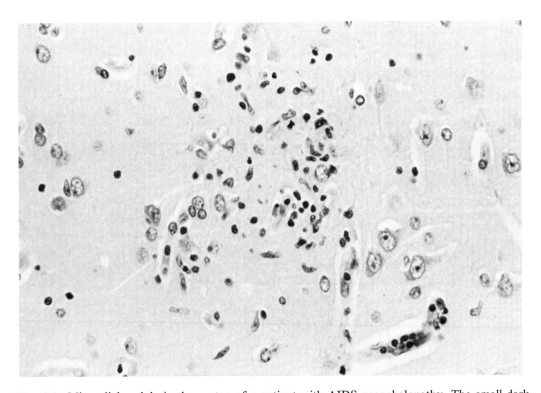

Fig. 3-1. Microglial nodule in the cortex of a patient with AIDS encephalopathy. The small dark nuclei clustered about the center of the section are microglial nuclei. The larger nuclei with prominent nucleoli are in neurons. Several capillaries with clear perivascular spaces run through the microscopic section. (Hematoxylin and eosin stain, original magnification ×250.)

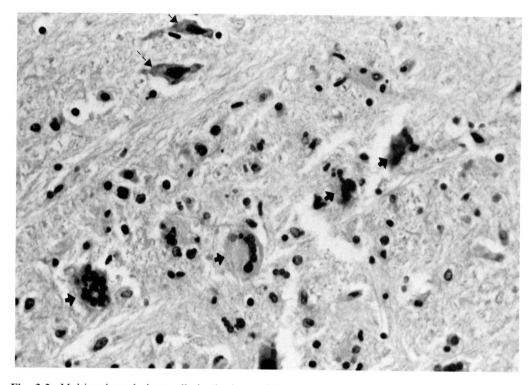

Fig. 3-2. Multinucleated giant cells in the base of the pons. Several multinucleated cells sit along the diagonal axis of this section through an area of microgliosis (arrows). At the top of the photomicrograph are two degenerating neurons lying parallel to each other with deeply staining, pyknotic nuclei (broken arrows). Neuronal death is not typical of AIDS encephalopathy, but giant cells and microglial nodules are. (Hematoxylin and eosin stain, original magnification ×400.)

these nodules, but multinucleated giant cells are routinely found in or near them. Some astrocytosis may also be evident with this pathologic change.

Microscopic examination of involved brain tissue consistently reveals gliosis, focal necrosis, atypical oligodendrocytes, and demyelination, as well as microglial nodules and multinucleated giant cells; but the degree to which any of these features is apparent is quite variable.[9,37,39,42] The multinucleated giant cells are among the most consistent findings in HIV encephalitis (Fig. 3-2). They appear to be derived from macrophages that have fused in response to HIV infection. These are also referred to as syncytial cells because they arise with the fusion of several individual cells, rather than from the duplication of nuclei in a transformed cell.

Demyelination may be prominent in some patients with HIV encephalopathy. The oligodendrocytes responsible for myelin formation are impaired in scattered areas throughout the brain. Oligodendrocytes often exhibit intracellular alterations, with nuclear enlargement appearing most commonly.[42] Axonal spheroids, indicative of axonal deterioration, occur along with the demyelination in patients with this subacute encephalitis.[37,39,42] Inflammatory changes associated with the demyelination are remarkably minor. A reactive astrocytosis may appear in some regions of this white matter. Cellular infiltrates, when they occur at all, are usually prominent in perivascular spaces and are limited to mononuclear cells and macrophages.

Although the cerebral hemispheres are often uniformly affected by this subacute encephalitis, there is significantly less disturbance of the brain stem, cerebellum, and spinal cord.[42] Areas in the brain that exhibit a slightly increased probability of having pathologic changes include the amygdala, hippocampus, putamen, frontal cortex, and temporal cortex.[42] The centrum semiovale also has a slightly greater probability of exhibiting encephalitis.[42] The cortical gray matter usually appears grossly intact, but microscopic studies show degenerating cells of different types scattered throughout the cerebral cortex.[9,16]

Some investigators have found that the severity of dementia exhibited by these patients correlates with the degree of cerebral involvement found at autopsy, but this correlation is fairly weak.[24,42] Others have described patients with profound dementia and relatively bland neuropathologic findings at autopsy.[7,39,40] Whether these discrepancies are caused by different strains of the virus or different neuropathologic mechanisms remains to be determined. There may, indeed, be HIV strains that preferentially replicate in the brain without causing substantial neurologic or immunologic disorders.[45] Such strains could cause a more insidious subacute encephalitis with less obvious neuropathologic findings.

Cells Infected by HIV

Human immunodeficiency virus has been identified in several cell types in the central nervous sysjtem.[9,16,20,32] All brain regions have evidence of the virus. Patients with the most severe form of the AIDS dementia complex have obvious viral antigen in predominantly subcortical regions.[9] The cells most clearly exhibiting evidence of HIV antigen, and therefore of viral infection, are monocytes, macrophages presumably de-

rived from these monocytes, and multinucleated giant cells derived from these macrophages.[9,10,11,16,32]

Viral antigen clearly occurs in acid-phosphatase-negative, process-bearing neuroglial cells, as well as in acid-phosphatase-positive cells of presumably endothelial origin.[9,47] That there is endothelial cell infection provides an alternative to the macrophage theory of HIV invasion of the central nervous system; rather than being carried in by infected macrophages, the virus could cross through the blood-brain barrier in sick endothelial cells.

The only neurons identified with HIV antigen intracellularly have been widely scattered and limited to the basal ganglia.[9,47] In fact, the extent to which neurons exhibit viral material indicates that they are incidental targets of infection, rather than the principal sites of HIV infection in the central nervous system. The proportion of neurons exhibiting HIV antigens or HIV proviral DNA is too small to account for the prominent neurologic disease exhibited by patients infected with the AIDS virus.

Multinucleated giant cell syncytia have HIV RNA readily demonstrable intracellularly.[11] Most of these heavily infected cells are near microglial nodules and in blood vessel walls or lumens.[16] The frequent association of microglial nodules and HIV antigens suggests that these histologic features may represent a localized immune response to HIV invasion.[16] The frontal, temporal, and parietal lobes are especially likely to have infected cells; and there is a rough correlation between the amount of HIV antigen apparent in the brain and the clinical severity of the subacute encephalitis.[16]

The multinucleated giant cell is the most heavily infected of the cell types exhibiting viral antigen.[9,11] Some of these cells are simply binucleate or trinucleate macrophages, but others are large globular cells with several nuclei displaced to the periphery.[9] Neuroglial cells, endothelial cells, and neurons are probably infected to a substantial degree only in the most severe cases.[9]

Cytotoxic-suppressor (CD8) T lymphocytes occur in foci of inflammation, but neither helper-inducer (CD4) T lymphocytes nor B lymphocytes can be found in these infected brains.[9] Aside from the multinucleated giant cells and microglial nodules, those features that appear most consistently in brains exhibiting this AIDS encephalitis are astrocytosis of the cerebral white matter and fibrillary gliosis of the cerebral gray matter[42] (see Table 3-6). These changes may occur in distinct patches or diffusely throughout the cerebral hemispheres.

Distinctive Features

The lesions seen in HIV subacute encephalitis are distinct from those occurring in toxoplasmosis, cytomegalovirus infection (CMV), and progressive multifocal leukoencephalopathy. The large necrotizing lesions typical of toxoplasmosis are not seen with this subacute encephalitis.[34] The ependymal and subependymal involvement typical of CMV, as well as the intranuclear inclusions typical of CMV, do not develop.[34] The oligodendrocytes with enlarged nuclei and amphophilic inclusions typical of progressive multifocal leukoencephalopathy are not found.[34] These distinctions are important because all of these other conditions may cause subacute encephalitis in patients with AIDS.

CASE HISTORY TWO. A 42-year-old Hispanic man was admitted after progressive intellectual deterioration that led to increasingly dangerous behavior, such as sleeping with a lighted cigarette in his mouth and leaving the stove on after cooking. His intellectual decline had been dismissed as a consequence of protracted alcohol abuse, but until 1 year before the admission he had been fastidious, sociable, and interested in politics. He had abused intravenous heroin and cocaine for several years until 5 years before the current admission.

During the first few months of the year before his admission, the patient stopped bathing, spoke and slept little, and wandered aimlessly. He began to drink continuously and displayed paranoid delusions. He frequently locked himself in the bathroom, armed with a knife. He lost about 50 pounds over the course of a year.

On examination at the time of his final admission he was emaciated, filthy, and disoriented to place, time, and situation. Profound psychomotor retardation was evident. He had auditory hallucinations and his remarks were tangential. Recent memory was impaired, and his attention span was short.

Computed tomography of the head revealed cerebral atrophy and enlarged ventricles.

Interstitial pneumonia developed shortly after his admission. Visual hallucinations developed and anxiety increased. He died during an episode of unexplained hypotension.

At autopsy, his brain exhibited changes consistent with AIDS encephalopathy (Fig. 3-3). The frontal and temporal white matter exhibited diffuse astrocytosis and microgliosis (Fig. 3-4). In both the frontal and temporal white matter, as well as in the brain stem, there were microglial nodules with multinucleated giant cells. The thalamus had neuronal dropout and gliosis, a finding presumably unrelated to the HIV-related subacute encephalitis.

HIV encephalitis was the dominant, if not the only, manifestation of HIV infection in this man throughout most of his illness. This disease was slowly progressive and unremitting, features typical of patients without complicating opportunistic infections. The terminal episode of hypotension may have been from autonomic dysfunction.

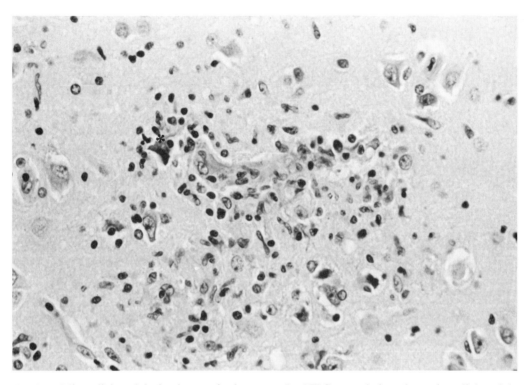

Fig. 3-3. Microglial nodule in the cerebral cortex. In AIDS encephalopathy, microglial nodules usually occur around or next to blood vessels, rather than in subpial or periventricular distributions. This microglial nodule with a multinucleated giant cell (*) was found on microscopic examination of the cerebral cortex. (Hematoxylin and eosin stain, original magnification ×250.)

PATHOPHYSIOLOGY

The principal route by which the human immunodeficiency virus enters and attacks the nervous system is still unknown. HIV can be isolated from the cerebrospinal fluid but it probably arrives there incidentally. The invasion of the brain and dissemination throughout the central nervous system is probably accomplished by virus carried into the central nervous system by infected macrophages and monocytes.[15,31,48] Macrophages and monocytes, as well as the multinucleated cells that form when they fuse with each other, contain most of the detectable HIV in the brains of AIDS victims.[28,31,49] Endothelial cell infection may also be important in the spread of the virus across the blood-brain barrier, but this is more controversial.[15]

Activation of the Virus

When infected macrophages or monocytes become activated or terminal differentiation occurs, the virus replicates.[50,51] Several different agents may activate a latent infection. These include infections with other viruses, but what combination of factors is necessary or sufficient for the activation of HIV in the central nervous system is unknown. That the infection may remain latent until a stimulus triggers it helps explain the variable interval observed be-

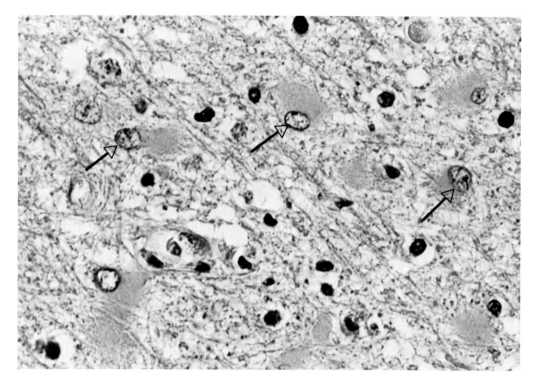

Fig. 3-4. Reactive astrocytosis in the white matter of a patient with AIDS encephalopathy. The astrocytes have large, pale-staining nuclei (arrows) sitting eccentrically at the margin of fairly homogeneous cytoplasmic material. The linear structures running primarily diagonally are myelin sheaths. (Hematoxylin and eosin stain, original magnification × 400.)

tween acquiring HIV and developing AIDS encephalopathy.

Because monocytes and macrophages can carry the virus in a latent form, they can survive long enough to migrate into the nervous system and spread the infection. The infected macrophages probably die after producing some of the virus, but before they die they may produce substances that are toxic to neural cells or incite local inflammatory cells that interfere with normal nerve cell function.[31,35] If they do not die, they will serve as persistent reservoirs of HIV. The fate of these cells is extremely important, since persistent infection in macrophages could pose an insurmountable barrier to antiviral therapies that are being developed to combat HIV.

Cellular Targets

How ever the virus arrives in the central nervous system, it exhibits an impressive affinity for a variety of cells in this type of tissue once it has arrived. In fact patients with HIV encephalopathy have more HIV RNA per infected cell in the brain than is observed in lymph nodes, peripheral blood, or bone marrow.[7] Unlike most retroviruses, the proviral DNA produced in brain tissue cells persists unintegrated into the DNA of the infected cells, a feature it shares with the visna virus, the retrovirus that causes a subacute encephalitis in sheep.[7] HIV is a cytopathic virus, and so it may be expected to kill the cells it infects at some point, although not necessarily early in the evolution of HIV encephalopathy.

Much of this outline of how HIV causes a subacute encephalitis is still speculative. Experimental studies show that the virus can infect glioma cell lines and human fetal brain cells. This does not mean that normal glial cells and mature neurons can be infected, but that is a possibility. Cell cultures that stain positively for glial fibrillary acidic protein (GFAP), a protein characteristic of astrocytes, get infected more easily than other glial cell cultures.[28] Cells that acquire the infection in the brain do not need to have the CD4 receptor typical of the helper-inducer (T4) lymphocyte, but some do appear to have this or a similar surface antigen.[28] In fact, dementia could evolve with no permanent damage to either glial cells or neurons if HIV caused endothelial damage alone. Viral damage to the endothelial cells of the brain capillaries would interfere with proper functioning of the blood-brain barrier and thereby undermine normal central nervous system function.[31] What the strategic cellular targets of HIV are remain undetermined, but what is evident is that nervous system dysfunction is not caused by neuronal loss.

Effects on Neurons

The invasion and destruction of neurons by HIV apparently does not play a significant role in the development of subacute encephalitis, but there are obvious indirect effects on neurons caused by viral infection of the central nervous system.[31] The virus or antigen associated with the virus may bind to vital receptor sites on neurons and nonneuronal CNS cells without causing infection and thereby disrupt normal function. A receptor similar to or identical with the CD4 receptor of T lymphocytes occurs on various glial cells in the brain and may normally bind endogenous peptides.[28] With viral binding to this site, binding of an essential agent, such as vasoactive intestinal peptide, could not occur.[28]

Membrane proteins and responses to various factors that are found in both the nervous system and the immune system may also be important in determining much of the neurologic disability and damage occurring with AIDS.[52] Neuroleukin, a neurotrophic factor that is produced by brain, as well as other organs, is structurally similar to part of the glycoprotein gp120 in the outermost coat of HIV.[31,35,52] This similarity may contribute to the effect on nervous system function exerted by the virus. With HIV or the gp120 component of HIV competing with neuroleukin, normal neuronal repair or growth might be impaired.[31,52,53] Even isolated from the rest of the virus, the glycoprotein gp120 of the AIDS virus coat can kill nonhuman nerve cells in culture.[53] Although HIV infects most cells by binding to the T4 (CD4) antigen on the target cell surface, the toxicity of the envelope glycoprotein gp120 appears to be independent of T4 antigen binding.[49,53] The cells affected in both the central and peripheral nervous system are neuroleukin-dependent neurons.[52] More than 60 percent of neuroleukin-dependent neurons die in the presence of gp120 in culture.[52] That this is part of the basis for the AIDS dementia complex remains to be established.

One of the most provocative features of neuroleukin is that it is a lymphokine: It is secreted by activated T lymphocytes and induces immunoglobulin secretion by mononuclear cells.[54] The viral coat protein gp120 interferes with the lymphokine activity of neuroleukin and may help suppress immune function in the AIDS patient at least partly by this mechanism.[52] What all this suggests is that the dementia evident in AIDS may be an incidental consequence of elements of the viral infection primarily directed against the immune system.[52]

HIV Envelope Activity

The HIV envelope glycoproteins may play several roles in the evolution and character of the encephalopathy that develops with the AIDS virus attack on the nervous system. The glycoprotein gp120 may be responsible for the relatively slight inflammatory response evident in AIDS encephalopathy. Gp120 stimulates human monocytes to release prostaglandins and leukotrienes.[53] One of the prostaglandins released, PGE2, is effective in damping the immune response, a response that would already be impaired by CD4 T lymphocyte depletion in AIDS.[53] Free gp120 also poses a danger for cells by making them targets for immune system attack when it binds to their surfaces.[53]

What gp120 of the viral envelope most certainly does is produce the multinucleated or syncytial cells characteristic of AIDS encephalopathy.[49] The expression of envelope glycoprotein on the surface of infected cells makes them fuse with other cells that have the CD4 (T4) receptor on their surfaces.[49] The CD4 receptor is the binding site for viral glycoprotein gp120.[49] Once gp120 is a component of the cell membrane, it induces fusion with other cell membranes that have the CD4 receptor. The syncytial cells that result are short-lived, but conspicuous in the central nervous system. Because they are a relatively short-lived product of HIV activation, their presence in the brain suggests that activation of latently infected cells occurs after they enter the nervous system. Indeed, the nervous system may be a favored site for HIV attack because it has substances that trigger the activation of latently infected cells.

TREATMENT POSSIBILITIES

There is no therapy effective against HIV subacute encephalitis. Zidovudine (AZT, Retrovir) may provide some relief from the inexorable progression of the disorder, but its long-term value against HIV damage to the nervous system remains to be demonstrated. Early reports on the effect of this antiviral agent on the progression of subacute encephalitis have been disappointing. Other antiviral agents, such as fusidic acid, are also likely to be ineffective because the encephalopathy appears to occur with relatively little viral replication. With aggressive treatment of associated infections, neurologic function will improve, but this should not be misconstrued as a substantial reversal of AIDS encephalopathy. Management of systemic and central nervous system disturbances developing during the evolution of HIV encephalopathy help to reduce the patient's incapacity.

The peculiar behavior of the retrovirus and its DNA provirus in the central nervous system increases the likelihood that an effective systemic treatment of HIV infection will fail to reverse disease in the central nervous system. Patients may be protected against acquired immune deficiency and be susceptible to progressive HIV encephalopathy. This poses the disturbing prospect that short-term treatments, such as zidovudine, may increase longevity without improving neurologic function. An enlarging population of AIDS patients would survive with dementia, spasticity, incontinence, ataxia, and seizures.

Myelopathy

Many of the patients with HIV encephalopathy have signs and symptoms of spinal cord disease.[30] In rare patients, this myelopathy is the dominant clinical problem. More than 20 percent of patients who die with AIDS have a myelopathy characterized by spongiform myelin changes in the dorsal and lateral columns of the spinal cord.[20,55] This is a vacuolar myelopathy (Fig. 3-5). There is damage to the myelin sheath in tracts of the spinal cord manifested by vacuolar changes in the myelin.[28] This lesion develops independently of any opportunistic infection and appears to be a direct consequence of HIV infection of the central nervous system.[32,42]

CLINICAL FINDINGS

Signs and symptoms of this vacuolar myelopathy include progressive paraparesis and spasticity.[55] Posterior column damage is manifest as impaired position and vibration sense. Additional problems routinely include gait ataxia and incontinence (Table 3-7). Deficits evolve over the course of weeks or months.[15] Patients with evident dementia have signs of myelopathy slightly more commonly than those with little or no dementia.[55] Presumably this is because HIV encephalitis and HIV myelitis worsen in concert.

DIAGNOSTIC STUDIES

Diagnostic studies are of limited usefulness in establishing the diagnosis. Myelography usually reveals a normal appearing spinal cord.[55] Autopsy studies demonstrate that the upper spinal cord is preferentially involved, but even this region appears normal on myelography.[42] Somatosensory evoked potential studies using nerves in the legs will exhibit nonspecific abnormalities. They will establish that there is probably a myelopathy, but they cannot discriminate among different causes for the myelopathy.

Table 3-7. Findings with Vacuolar Myelopathy

Clinical	Pathologic
Progressive spastic paraparesis	Demyelination
	Vacuolation of lateral
Impaired vibration and position sense	and posterior columns
	Foamy macrophages
Gait ataxia	Reactive microglial cells
Incontinence	and astrocytes
	Rare microglial nodules

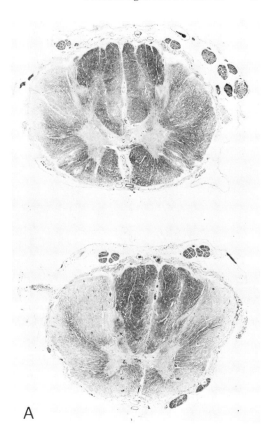

A

Fig. 3-5. AIDS myelopathy. (**A**) Cross-sections of the thoracic spinal cord in a patient with AIDS myelopathy were stained for myelin. There is prominent vacuolation and loss of myelin, which is most severe in the lateral columns. (Weil stain for myelin ×6.) (*Figure continues.*)

If the patient also has a neuropathy along with the spinal cord disease, the evoked potential studies will not be able to demonstrate the myelopathy. The resolution of magnetic resonance is still too poor to unequivocally reveal the myelin changes associated with this vacuolar myelopathy. Computed tomography is even less useful.

HISTOPATHOLOGY

Vacuolar changes in the affected spinal cords are usually most prominent in the posterior and lateral columns.[42] The lateral col-

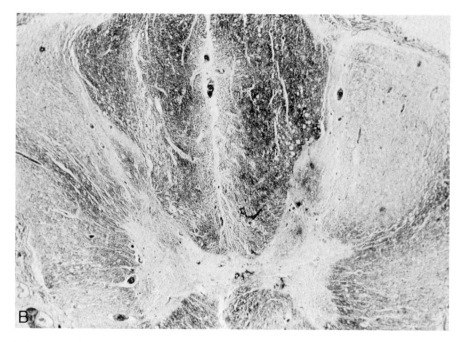

Fig. 3-5. (*continued*) (**B**) Low-power view of the thoracic cord shows vacuolation in the posterior and lateral columns and loss of myelin in the lateral columns. (Weil stain for myelin, × 17.)

umns are more severely affected than the posterior columns and the gray matter is largely unaffected.[55] Where vacuolation is most prominent, there is little or no evidence of inflammation; strictly spongiform changes occur in the parenchyma of the spinal cord and anterior horn cells are spared.[32,42] Some macrophages may be found in regions with extensive myelin damage, and associated axonal damage may be manifest as axonal spheroids on histologic studies.[55]

The spongiform appearance of the cord is from vacuolar swelling within the myelin sheaths of dorsal and lateral white matter[55] (Fig. 3-6). Fluid accumulates between discrete layers of myelin and may dissect away part of the myelin sheath surrounding the nerve fiber, without actually fragmenting the myelin. Damage to the myelin extends beyond the cord proper and affects spinal roots (Fig. 3-7). Although there is consid-erable speculation that HIV directly invades neural elements in the spinal cord, no virus has yet been convincingly isolated from nonlymphoid cells in the spinal cord.[32]

Case History Three

A 40-year-old black man with a history of intravenous drug and alcohol abuse was admitted with leg weakness. He believed that he had problems with both of his lower legs over the course of 9 months. During the month before his admission, this problem had progressed sufficiently to interfere with gait and bladder control.

Past problems had included endocarditis. His intellectual function was relatively good, and no cranial nerve deficits were evident. Arm strength was good and sensation was largely preserved in the legs. Leg strength was diffusely impaired in all major

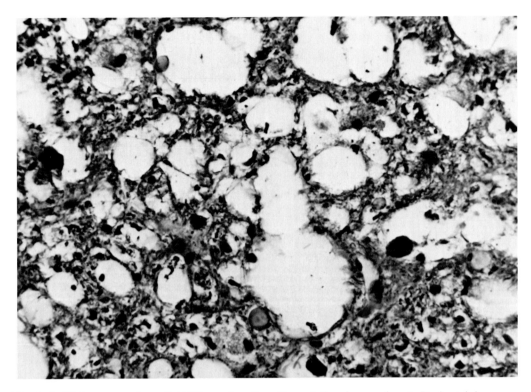

Fig. 3-6. High power view of AIDS myelopathy. Vacuolation is prominent. Dark staining axons are displaced to the edges of the vacuoles. (Bodian stain, original magnification ×250.)

groups of both legs. He could just overcome gravity with exertion. There was symmetric hyperreflexia in the legs, and clonus was evident at the ankles. A myelogram revealed no structural problems overlying the cord, but the cerebrospinal fluid protein was 81 mg/dL. There were 9 red blood cells/μL and 14 white blood cells/μL, all of which were lymphocytes.

While smoking in bed, the patient sustained burns on his right arm. He subsequently developed oral candidiasis. A repeat spinal tap revealed persistent elevation of the CSF white blood cell count to 15 cells/μL. Computed tomography and MRI of the brain revealed atrophy, but no focal lesions. He developed persistent fevers with consistently negative blood and urine cultures. His leg strength showed progressive deterioration, and bilaterally positive Babinski

signs developed. His cognitive function deteriorated progressively and he developed generalized seizures. Within 2 months of the admission for paraparesis, the patient was grossly paraplegic. He expired without ever showing recovery of leg strength or bladder control.

Autopsy revealed changes typical of AIDS encephalomyelopathy. These included perivascular microglial nodules with multinucleated giant cells in the cerebral and cerebellar white matter, as well as in the basal ganglia, brain stem, and spinal cord. A vacuolar myelopathy was evident, with extensive vacuolar changes in the myelin sheaths along tracts in the cervical, thoracic, and lumbar segments of the spinal cord. The lateral columns were most damaged, but vacuolation was evident in the anterior and posterior columns as well.

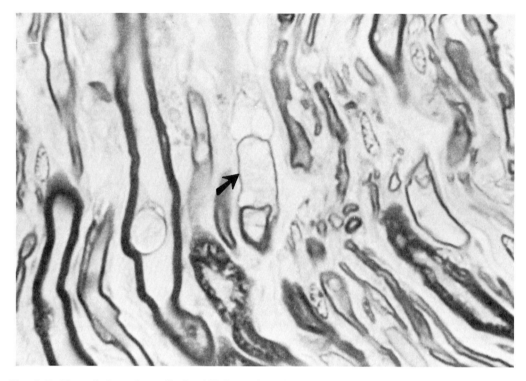

Fig. 3-7. Vacuolation of myelin in AIDS myelopathy. That vacuole formation occurs between individual layers of myelin is evident in the myelin sheath in the center of this section, which is split to surround an "intramyelinic" vacuole (arrow). (Toluidine blue stain, original magnification ×400.)

Luxol fast blue stain showed extensive loss of myelin, mainly in the lateral columns, associated with the vacuolization. The vacuolated white matter also contained foamy macrophages and a few reactive microglial cells and astrocytes. Vacuolar changes were apparent even in the nerve roots. A few microglial nodules without multinucleated cells were evident in the sacral gray matter. In peripheral nerves, there was mild swelling of some segments of myelin sheath, but there were no foamy macrophages or other inflammatory cell infiltrates.

Spinal cord disease was the initial and principal manifestation of this patient's HIV infection. The encephalopathy that subsequently developed was always overshadowed by his paraplegia, even though the autopsy examination revealed problems in the brain, as well as the spinal cord.

PATHOPHYSIOLOGY

Vacuolar myelopathy may be caused by direct infection of the spinal cord oligodendrocytes by the AIDS virus, but evidence that the AIDS virus actually enters and infects spinal cord glial cells is still weak.[28] Some investigators believe that they have evidence of mature virions budding from infected glial cells, with oligodendrocytes more often affected than astrocytes.[28] The virus is presumed to gain access to the spinal cord by the same routes used in HIV encephalopathy, that is, primarily within infected macrophages or monocytes or across infected endothelial cells.[8,30]

Some patients have rapid deterioration of spinal cord function, but others remain largely asymptomatic. Why spinal cord deterioration is especially prominent in some patients is unknown, but it is probably related to preexisting spinal cord disease. The diseased cord quickly becomes symptomatic because compensatory mechanisms are limited. There are no measures that affect the course or outcome of this vacuolar myelopathy.

Aseptic Meningitis

An additional central nervous system problem that may occur early with HIV infection is aseptic meningitis.[15] Relatively few patients have substantial evidence of this meningitis, but those who do develop it usually exhibit signs and symptoms soon after they develop detectable HIV antibodies in their serum.[56] The true prevalence of this condition has not yet been defined because it has been looked for infrequently in the general population of AIDS victims. This is a self-limited condition, during which HIV can be isolated from the blood and cerebrospinal fluid of affected individuals.[57] Why it often occurs before other signs or symptoms of nervous system disease is unknown.

Affected patients complain of headache, photophobia, malaise, myalgias, and arthralgias. On examination they often have fever and neck stiffness. Occasionally a rash is evident.[56] Cranial nerves V, VII, and VIII may be impaired during the acute meningitis.[27] The CSF findings are typical of those seen with aseptic meningitis. There is usually a low-grade pleocytosis, with up to a few hundred WBCs/μL, most of which are mononuclear cells.[57] Spinal fluid proteins may be greatly increased to as high as 1 g/dL.[27,57] The glucose content is not usually significantly depressed.

The aseptic meningitis caused by HIV resolves spontaneously within days in most cases. In a few cases, the condition has been more chronic, and in rare cases it has been recurrent.[58] Aseptic meningitis has no prognostic value since patients may develop subacute encephalitis either quickly or after a substantial delay once the meningitis has been diagnosed.

Peripheral Nervous System Disease

Nervous system disease with AIDS is not limited to the central nervous system. In some individuals, demyelinating peripheral neuropathy associated with HIV infection may produce the only neurologic symptoms associated with the infection.[59,60] Autopsy and biopsy studies indicate that more than 90 percent of patients with AIDS develop some form of peripheral neuropathy and at least half of these have complaints directly attributable to the neuropathy.[61] Most commonly the patient has sensory or motor disturbances, but at least 10 percent of patients have autonomic problems, such as orthostatic hypotension.[61]

Both sensory and motor nerve problems occurring in patients with AIDS may be the direct effects of HIV infection or the effects of an as yet unidentified opportunistic infection.[27,59,62,63] Although some of the viruses producing neurologic disease in AIDS, such as varicella-zoster, may produce a neuropathy, there evidently are many cases of neuropathy caused by HIV itself. The AIDS virus, HIV-1, has been cultured from nerves in affected individuals.[58]

CLINICAL FINDINGS

The peripheral neuropathy may take one of several forms. The most common is a symmetric, distal sensory polyneuropathy. Patients with this progressive neuropathy usually complain of painful, burning dyses-thesias symmetrically; distal sensory prob-lems are more prominent than weak-ness.[27,60] If weakness does occur, it is often associated with atrophy.[27]

Alternatively, the patient may have a mononeuritis multiplex or a chronic inflam-matory demyelinating polyneuropathy sim-ilar to Guillain-Barré syndrome.[15] This polyradiculopathy may resolve at the same pace as HIV-unrelated Guillain-Barré syn-dromes or may be one of many neurologic problems that appear and persist in the pa-tient with HIV infection. This chronic polyneuropathy occasionally develops be-fore the appearance of other signs of AIDS and may resolve spontaneously.[22,60] Some patients develop combinations of problems, such as a chronic inflammatory polyneu-ropathy with mononeuritis multiplex or an asymmetric distal neuropathy.[22,60]

It is fairly common for some type of pe-ripheral neuropathy to develop in patients with HIV encephalomyelitis. These pa-tients have demyelination in their periph-eral nerves with sparing of the axons in 50 percent of specimens obtained at the time of autopsy.[42] The peripheral neuropathy in these patients may be masked by the symp-toms associated with the central nervous system disease.

Case History Four

A 50-year-old homosexual man devel-oped left shoulder weakness and atrophy over the course of a few weeks. Treatment with prednisone had no effect on the prob-lem, and the deficits persisted unchanged for several months. Five months after the first weakness developed in the shoulder, he noticed progressive numbness on the soles of both of his feet. This extended onto his legs in a stocking distribution over the course of a few weeks. No other deficits developed.

Before the appearance of the weakness and numbness, the patient had no signifi-cant illnesses. A minor cellulitis, appearing 6 months before his neurologic complaints began, cleared quickly with oral antibiotic treatment. Shortly thereafter an enlarged lymph node from his axilla was biopsied. It revealed proliferative changes consistent with, but not diagnostic of, AIDS.

One month after his weakness appeared a serum protein electrophoresis revealed a polyclonal elevation of his gamma globulins to more than twice the normal level (Fig. 3-8). A computed tomogram of the shoulder and an MRI of the spine were both unre-vealing.

Six months after the appearance of shoul-der weakness, lymphocyte studies were performed. These revealed a depression of the CD4 T lymphocyte count to 639/μL and elevation of the CD8 T lymphocyte count to 968/μL. The CD4/CD8 ratio was inverted to 0.65. EMG and nerve conduction studies revealed changes consistent with a demye-linating, peripheral neuropathy, unasso-ciated with myopathy.

This patient was presumed to have an HIV mononeuritis multiplex in combination with a distal sensory neuropathy. He had no other significant deficits despite his poor hematologic picture. Several months after the hematologic studies were completed, he continued to have no evidence of oppor-tunistic infections or dementia.

DIAGNOSTIC STUDIES

Patients with any of the HIV related pe-ripheral neuropathies or radiculopathies ex-hibit characteristic changes on objective tests (Table 3-8). Electrodiagnostic tests re-veal slowed nerve conduction velocities and some conduction blocks.[62] Sensory and motor compound action potentials are usu-ally of low amplitude.[60] Early in the course of peripheral nerve damage, the electrodi-agnostic picture is consistent with primary demyelination, but later in the disease there

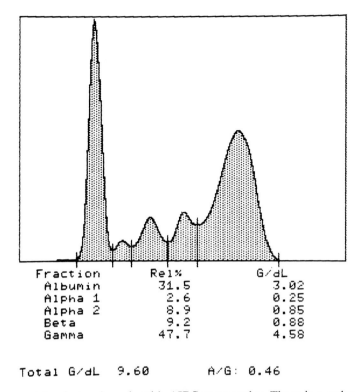

Fraction	Rel%	G/dL
Albumin	31.5	3.02
Alpha 1	2.6	0.25
Alpha 2	8.9	0.85
Beta	9.2	0.88
Gamma	47.7	4.58

Total G/dL 9.60   A/G: 0.46

Fig. 3-8. Serum protein electrophoresis with AIDS neuropathy. There is a polyclonal increase in the gamma globulin fraction of the serum proteins.

is secondary axonal loss.[59] The cerebrospinal fluid protein is greater than 200 mg/dl in many of the patients with neuropathy or radiculopathy, but this may be from asymptomatic central nervous system disease.[59,62] The mononuclear cell content of the cerebrospinal fluid is also usually elevated, but the mean cell count is less than 23 mononuclear cells/μL.[59] The CSF IgG is characteristically elevated, and antibodies to HIV can be detected in the CSF.[62]

Table 3-8. AIDS Neuropathy

Clinical Signs	Microscopic Findings
Sensory and motor signs	Segmental demyelination
Autonomic dysfunction	Mild axonal loss
Slow nerve conduction velocities	Mononuclear infiltrates
Conduction blocks	Intra-axonal particulate inclusions
Desynchronized evoked responses	
Elevated CSF protein content	
Elevated CSF IgG	
HIV antibody titers measurable in the CSF	

HISTOPATHOLOGY

Sural nerve biopsy performed on AIDS patients with symptomatic neuropathy often reveals segmental demyelination, axonal loss, and mononuclear infiltrates in the epineurium or endoneurium.[59,62] Endoneurial edema may be substantial.[60] The demyelination is laminar in character and involves many axons, at least in a sensory nerve like the sural nerve[62,63] (Fig. 3-9). Along with the demyelination, there is ax-

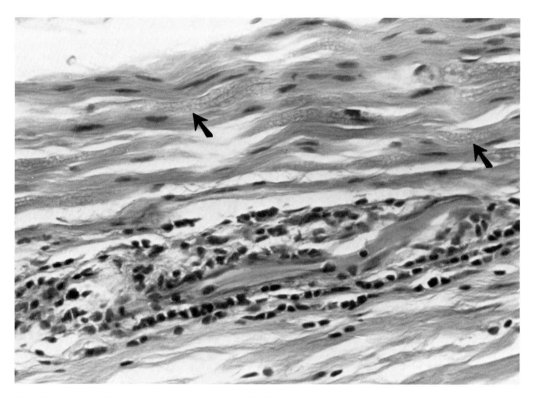

Fig. 3-9. Longitudinal section of nerve in AIDS neuropathy. Considerable fibrosis and loss of myelin is apparent. Remaining myelinated fibers appear as narrow, interrupted strips of foamy material (arrows), most evident in the upper half of the section and separated by fibrous tissue. There is also a perivascular mononuclear cell infiltrate in the lower half of the section. (Hematoxylin and eosin stain, original magnification ×250.)

onal damage and fibrosis (Plate 3-1). Occasionally, the perineurial cells have prominent vacuolation, reminiscent of the vacuolar changes seen in HIV myelopathy, but this is a distinctly inconsistent finding in peripheral nerve specimens.[59] The mononuclear infiltrate consists of CD8 cytotoxic-suppressor lymphocytes and macrophages.[61] Vasculitis associated with demyelinating neuropathy may be evident (Plate 3-2).

What appear to be virus particles have been found on electron microscopic examination of axons, but not in Schwann cells of peripheral nerves.[62] If the retrovirus is present in the axon, a mechanism for transporting the viral material from the nerve cell body would need to be postulated.[62] There are no ribosomes in the axon, and ribosomes are essential for the manufacture of the viral RNA.[62]

TREATMENT

This HIV-related neuropathy and radiculopathy has been treated with plasmapheresis and prednisone therapy with encouraging results in some cases, but many patients exhibit spontaneously remitting and relapsing courses.[59,60] In fact, most of the patients studied have had remarkably good recoveries from this neuropathy regardless of treatment.[59] Establishing whether any treatment is useful is impossible with the few cases studied to date.

MUSCLE DISEASE

Patients with AIDS occasionally develop a polymyositis that has no apparent source other than the HIV infection.[27,63,64] In rare patients, this polymyositis may be the first manifestation of an HIV infection.[64] These patients exhibit progressive proximal or distal muscle weakness, face and neck muscle weakness, and markedly elevated creatine phosphokinase.[33] Occasionally the weakness is strictly distal and the creatine phosphokinase is normal, but such features are atypical for a viral polymyositis.[63]

Symptoms of the myositis include leg cramps, muscle tenderness, and weakness.[1] Atrophy may be evident in severely affected muscles.[63] The electromyogram exhibits denervation, as well as characteristic myopathic changes, such as increased insertional activity and bizarre high frequency discharges.[33,63]

Microscopic examination of the affected muscles reveals fiber necrosis with variations in fiber size and central rod bodies in the fibers of some patients.[33] Inflammatory infiltrates occur in most patients but are not invariably present[33] (Fig. 3-10). Multinucleated giant cells are obvious in some patients

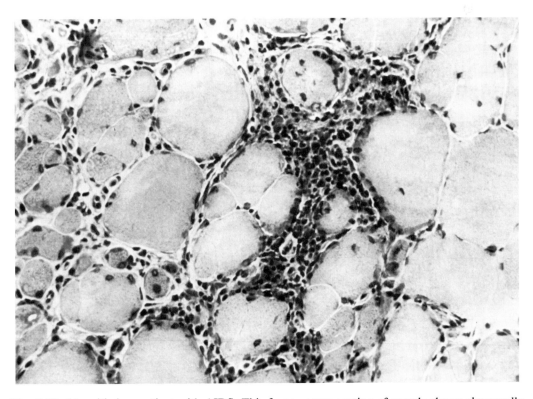

Fig. 3-10. Myositis in a patient with AIDS. This frozen cross section of muscle shows abnormally small muscle fibers intermixed with fibers of normal size. Some of the small fibers are regenerating, as indicated by their large and occasionally internally displaced nuclei. There is an extensive inflammatory infiltrate between the muscle fibers within this fascicle, of the sort seen in myositis. (Hematoxylin and eosin stain, original magnification ×250.)

who do have an inflammatory infiltrate, and this histologic feature has been considered evidence that the HIV is directly responsible for the myositis.[63] Multinucleated giant cells are typical of granulomatous inflammations, rather than viral myopathies, and so the appearance of these cells in the muscles affected suggests an atypical viral infection.[63] Because the type of giant cell seen is identical to that occurring in the central nervous system with HIV subacute encephalitis, it may, in fact, be a histologic marker of the disease when it occurs in association with polymyositis.

No viral particles have been observed in affected muscles. Cultures of inflamed muscle have yet to yield HIV, but immunocytochemical studies in a few patients have demonstrated reactivity of the inflammatory infiltrates with anti-HIV antiserum.[64] HIV antigens have been found in CD4-positive lymphoid cells in the infiltrate about the muscle fibers and invading the endomysial septa.[64] Patients with this type of polymyositis are likely to exhibit considerable evidence of peripheral neuropathy.[63] As is typical of myopathies associated with other neuropathies, fiber type grouping is occasionally seen.[63]

Treatment with azathioprine and prednisone may be useful, but no controlled or protracted studies have been performed.[33] Some patients exhibit considerable improvement with conventional anti-inflammatory drugs.[63] Some have resolution of the myositis without any treatment at all.[65]

CEREBROVASCULAR COMPLICATIONS

Common neurologic problems may develop in uncommon ways in patients with AIDS. Patients with this syndrome are at increased risk of nonbacterial thrombotic endocarditis which in turn will produce embolic strokes.[1] Subarachnoid and intracerebral hemorrhages occur in association with the thrombocytopenia that develops in many patients with AIDS.[66–68] Thrombocytopenia occurs because platelets are destroyed at an inordinately high rate in the peripheral blood, not because production is decreased.[66] This excessive turnover in platelets appears to have an autoimmune basis.[66]

Cerebrovascular accidents for less obvious reasons have also occurred in patients with AIDS. Infarction may develop with fungal infections, such as cryptococcosis, as well as with other opportunistic infections.[66] In rare individuals, intracerebral hemorrhages have developed in metastatic nodules of Kaposi's sarcoma.[22] Nonhemorrhagic infarctions have been ascribed to Herpes zoster arteritis in some individuals, but this is difficult to establish.[22]

Granulomatous angiitis has also been described in a patient with HIV infection.[69] Pathologic features of this cerebral angiitis include fibrous intimal thickening in intracranial blood vessels and transmural mononuclear cell infiltrates.[69] Multinucleated giant cells are evident adjacent to the internal elastic lamina, and involved blood vessels have segmental narrowing apparent on routine angiography.[69] Involved blood vessels develop thrombosis with intraluminal occlusion.[69] This angiitis may actually result from an opportunistic viral infection, rather than from HIV infection directly, but its etiology remains unknown.[69]

As AIDS becomes more common, it will account for an increasing proportion of the cerebrovascular accidents occurring in young people. The routine investigation of any young person with a cerebrovascular accident must include an assessment of the patient's immune status and HIV seropositivity. Thrombocytopenia, granulomatous angiitis, and intracerebral hemorrhages cannot be considered idiopathic until HIV infection has been disproved. Precautions must be taken with any young person developing cerebrovascular occlusion or hemorrhage until it has been established that HIV is not responsible.

REFERENCES

1. Berger JR, Moskowitz L, Fischl M, Kelley RE: Neurologic disease as the presenting manifestation of acquired immunodeficiency syndrome. South Med J 80:683, 1987
2. Britton CB, Miller JR: Neurologic complications in acquired immunodeficiency syndrome (AIDS). Neurol Clin 2:315, 1984
3. Anders KH, Guerra WF, Tomiyasu U, et al: The neuropathology of AIDS. UCLA experience and review. Am J Pathol 124:537, 1986
4. Anders KH, Steinsapir KD, Iverson DJ, et al: Neuropathologic findings in the acquired immunodeficiency syndrome (AIDS). Clin Neuropathol 5:1, 1986
5. Herman P: Neurologic complications of acquired immunologic deficiency syndrome. Neurology, 33:suppl. 2, 105, 1983
6. Koppel BS, Wormser GP, Tuchman AJ, et al: Central nervous system involvement in patients with acquired immunodeficiency syndrome. Acta Neurol Scand 71:337, 1985
7. Shaw GM, Harper ME, Hahn BH, et al: HTLV-III infection in brains of children and adults with AIDS encephalopathy. Science 227:177, 1985
8. Ho DD, Rota TR, Hirsch MS: Infection of monocyte/macrophages by human T lymphotropic virus type III. J Clin Invest 77:1712, 1986
9. Pumarola-Sune T, Navia BA, Cordon-Cardo C, et al: HIV antigen in the brains of patients with the AIDS dementia complex. Ann Neurol 21:490, 1987
10. Gartner S, Markovits P, Markovits DM, et al: Virus isolation from and identification of HTLV-III/LAV-producing cells in brain tissue from a patient with AIDS. JAMA 256:2365, 1986
11. Koyanagi Y, Miles S, Mitsuyasu RT, et al: Dual infection of the central nervous system by AIDS viruses with distinct cellular tropisms. Science 236:819, 1987
12. Koenig S, Gendelman HE, Orenstein JM, et al: Detection of AIDS virus in macrophages in brain tissue from AIDS patients with encephalopathy. Science 233:1089, 1986
13. Sharer LR, Cho E-S, Epstein LG: Multinucleated giant cells and HTLV-III in AIDS encephalopathy. Hum Pathol 16:760, 1986
14. Sharer LR, Kapila R: Neuropathologic observations in the acquired immunodeficiency syndrome. Acta Neuropathol 66:188, 1985
15. Gabuzda DH, Hirsch MS: Neurologic manifestations of infection with human immunodeficiency virus. Ann Intern Med 107:383, 1987
16. Gabuzda DH, Ho DD, de la Monte SM, et al: Immunohistochemical identification of HTLV-III antigen in brains of patients with AIDS. Ann Neurol 20:289, 1986
17. FDA: Special AIDS issue. FDA Drug Bull 17:14, 1987
18. CDC: Revision of the CDC surveillance case definition for acquired immunodeficiency syndrome. MMWR 36:3s, 1987
19. Johnson RT: Viral Infections of the Nervous System. Raven Press, New York, 1982
20. Roman GC: Retrovirus-associated myelopathies. Arch Neurol 44:659, 1987
21. Faulstich ME: Psychiatric aspects of AIDS. Am J Psychiatry 1444:551, 1987
22. Levy RM, Bredesen DE, Rosenblum ML: Neurologic manifestations of the acquired immunodeficiency syndrome (AIDS): Experience at the University of California at San Francisco and review of the literature. J Neurosurg 62:475, 1985
23. Hoffman RS: Neuropsychiatric complications of AIDS. Psychosomatics 25:393, 1984
24. Faulstich ME: Acquired immune deficiency syndrome: an overview of central nervous system complications and neuropsychological sequelae. Int J Neurosci 30:249, 1986
25. Navia BA, Price RW: The acquired immunodeficiency syndrome dementia complex as the presenting or sole manifestation of human immunodeficiency virus infection. Arch Neurol 44:65, 1987
26. Nielson SL, Petito CK, Urmacher CD, Posner JB: Subacute encephalitis in acquired immune deficiency syndrome: a postmortem study. Am J Clin Pathol 82:678, 1984
27. Snider WD, Simpson DM, Nielsen S, et al: Neurological complications of acquired immune deficiency syndrome: analysis of 50 patients. Ann Neurol 14:408, 1983
28. Barnes DM: Brain damage by AIDS under active study. Science 235:1574, 1987
29. Koenig S, Gendelman HE, DalCanto MC, et al: Detection of AIDS retroviral RNA in

nonlymphoid cells in the brain of an AIDS patient with encephalopathy. Clinical Research 34:722A, 1986

30. Sharer LR, Epstein LG, Cho ES, Petito CK: HTLV-III and vacuolar myelopathy of AIDS. N Engl J Med 315:62, 1986

31. Ho DD, Pomerantz RJ, Kaplan JC: Pathogenesis of infection with human immunodeficiency virus. N Engl J Med 317:278, 1987

32. Johnson RT, McArthur JC: Myelopathies and retroviral infections. Ann Neurol 21:113, 1987

33. Simpson DM, Bender AN: HTLV-III-associated myopathy. Neurology, 37:suppl. 1, 319, 1987

34. Barnes DM: Debate over potential AIDS drug. Science 237:128, 1987

35. Edwards DD: 'Competition' cause of AIDS dementia? Science News 132:150, 1987

36. Anand R, Siegal F, Reed C, et al: Noncytocidal natural variants of human immunodeficiency virus isolated from AIDS patients with neurological disorders. Lancet 2:234, 1987

37. Navia BA, Jordan BD, Price RW: The AIDS dementia complex: I. Clinical features. Ann Neurol 19:517, 1986

38. Navia BA, Jordan BD, Price RW: The AIDS dementia complex: II. Neuropathology, Ann Neurol 19:525, 1986

39. Vinters HV: The AIDS dementia complex. Ann Neurol 21:612, 1987

40. Navia BA, Cho E-S, Petito CK, Price RW: The AIDS dementia complex. Reply. Ann Neurol 21:612, 1987

41. Kaslow RA, Phair JP, Freidman HB, et al: Infection with human immunodeficiency virus: clinical manifestations and their relationship to immune deficiency. Ann Intern Med 107:474, 1987

42. de la Monte SM, Ho DD, Schooley RT, et al: Subacute encephalomyelitis of AIDS and its relation to HTLV-III infection. Neurology 37:562, 1987

43. Nath JA, Jancovic J, Pettigrew LC: Movement disorders and AIDS. Neurology 37:37, 1987

44. Metzer WS: Movement disorders with AIDS encephalopathy: case report. Neurology 37:1438, 1987

45. Hollander HR, Levy JA: Neurologic abnormalities and recovery of human immunodeficiency virus from cerebrospinal fluid. Ann Intern Med 106:692, 1987

46. Epstein LG, Sharer LR, Cho E-S, et al: HTLV-III/LAV-like retrovirus particles in the brains of patients with AIDS encephalopathy. AIDS Research 1:447, 1985

47. Wiley CA, Schrier RD, Nelson JA, et al: Cellular localization of human immunodeficiency virus infection within the brains of acquired immunodeficiency syndrome (AIDS) patients. Proc Natl Acad Sci USA 83:7089, 1986

48. Haase AT: Pathogenesis of lentivirus infections. Nature 322:130, 1986

49. Kowalski M, Potz J, Basiripour L, et al: Functional regions of the envelope glycoprotein of human immunodeficiency virus type 1. Science 237:1351, 1987

50. Gendelman HE, Narayan O, Kennedy-Stoskopf S, et al: Tropism of sheep lentiviruses for monocytes: susceptibility to infection and virus gene expression increases during maturation of monocytes to macrophages. J Virol 58:67, 1986

51. Barnes DM: Cytokines alter AIDs virus production. Science 236:1627, 1987

52. Lee MR, Ho DR, Gurney ME: Functional interaction and partial homology between human immunodeficiency virus and neuroleukin. Science 237:1047, 1987

53. Barnes DM: Solo actions of AIDS virus coat. Science 237:971, 1987

54. Gurney ME, Heinrich SA, Lee MR, Yin H-S: Molecular cloning and expression of neuroleukin, a neurotrophic factor for spinal and sensory neurons. Science 235:566, 1986

55. Petito CK, Navia BA, Cho ES, et al: Vacuolar myelopathy pathologically resembling subacute combined degeneration in patients with the acquired immunodeficiency syndrome. N Engl J Med 312:874, 1985

56. Cooper DA, Gold J, Maclean P, et al: Acute AIDS retrovirus infection: definition of a clinical illness associated with seroconversion. Lancet 1:537–540, 1985

57. Ho DD, Sarngadharan MG, Resnick L, et al: Primary human T-lymphotropic virus type III infection. Ann Intern Med 103:880, 1985

58. Ho DD, Rota TR, Schooley RT, et al: Isolation of HTLV-III from cerebrospinal fluid

and neural tissue of patients with neurologic syndromes related to the acquired immunodeficiency syndrome. N Engl J Med 313:1493, 1985

59. Cornblath DR, McArthur JC, Kennedy PGE, et al: Inflammatory demyelinating peripheral neuropathies associated with human T-cell lymphotropic virus type III infection. Ann Neurol 21:32, 1987

60. Lipkin WI, Parry G, Kiprov D, Abrams D: Inflammatory neuropathy in homosexual men with lymphadenopathy. Neurology 35:1479, 1985

61. de la Monte SM, Gabuzda DH, Ho DD, et al: Peripheral neuropathy in the acquired immune deficiency syndrome [Abstract]. Lab Invest 56:17A, 1987

62. Bailey RO, Singh JK, Bishop MB: AIDS neuropathy: the role of axoplasmic transport. Neurology, 37:suppl. 1, 356, 1987

63. Bailey RO, Turok DI, Jaufmann BP, Singh JK: Myositis and acquired immunodeficiency syndrome. Hum Pathol 18:749, 1987

64. Dalakas MC, Pezeshkpour GH, Gravell M, Sever JL: Polymyositis associated with AIDS retrovirus. JAMA 256:2381, 1986

65. Snider WD, Simpson DM, Aronyk KE, Nielsen SL: Primary lymphoma of the nervous system associated with acquired immune-deficiency syndrome. N Engl J Med 308:45, 1983

66. Desforges J, Mark EJ: Case record 41-1987. N Engl J Med 317:946, 1987

67. Abrams DI, Kiprov DD, Goedert JJ, et al: Antibodies to human T-lymphotropic virus type III and development of acquired immune deficiency syndrome in homosexual men presenting with immune thrombocytopenia. Ann Intern Med 104:47, 1986

68. Morris L, Distenfeld A, Amorosi E, Karpatkin S: Autoimmune thrombocytopenic purpura in homosexual men. Ann Intern Med 96:714, 1982

69. Yankner BA, Skolnik PR, Shoukimas GM, et al: Cerebral granulomatous angiitis associated with isolation of human T lymphotropic virus type III from the central nervous system. Ann Neurol 20:362, 1986

4

Opportunistic Infections

Patients with the acquired immune deficiency syndrome (AIDS) invariably develop opportunistic infections, that is, infections not usually occurring in or not lethal to individuals with intact immune systems. The organisms responsible for the nervous system infections in patients with AIDS include many routinely seen in immunocompromised patients without AIDS.[1-6] Unfortunately, the spectrum of opportunistic infections attacking the nervous system of the patient with AIDS is not entirely the same as that previously encountered in patients with drug-induced immunosuppression and other causes of immune deficiency[2,6-9] (Table 4-1). In addition, the response of the nervous system in the patient with AIDS is not the same as that in patients immunocompromised by drugs, lymphomas, leukemias, or genetic defects. Consequently, much of the experience with the natural history and treatment of opportunistic infections in immunocompromised patients without AIDS is not accurate or useful in the management of patients with AIDS.

The nervous system disease most often proving fatal in individuals with AIDS is *Toxoplasma gondii* encephalitis, but lethal central nervous system infections from cryptococcus, nocardia, cytomegalovirus, and nontuberculous mycobacteria are also common.[1,7-9] Some of the infections that occur in the nervous system of patients with AIDS are not strictly opportunistic, but they develop more commonly and are more resistant to treatment in the immunodeficient patient. Conventional causes of life-threatening meningoencephalitis, such as herpes simplex type 1 and tuberculosis, occur in patients with AIDS, although less commonly than truly opportunistic infections. Neurosyphilis in its varied forms is also somewhat opportunistic in the AIDS patient in that it evolves much more rapidly and perniciously than is encountered with conventional *Treponema pallidum* infections.[10]

Many of the viruses that cause substantial neurologic problems in patients with AIDS belong to the herpesvirus group.[11,12] These include herpes simplex (HSV) type 1 and 2, cytomegalovirus (CMV), varicella-zoster (VZV), and Epstein-Barr (EBV). All of these viruses are usually cell associated and have a propensity to assume a latent state.[11] Precisely why herpesviruses are especially troublesome in AIDS patients is not known. One possibility is that the latent viruses reside in lymphocytes and are activated when the immune system is injured by HIV.

Although the infectious agents most often responsible for neurologic disease in AIDS patients cause dysfunction by directly invading the neural tissues, they occasionally produce problems less directly. In some immunodeficient individuals, neurologic signs develop from focal lesions, such as an

Table 4-1. Common Opportunistic Infections
Affecting the Nervous System[a]

AIDS Patients	Immunosuppressed Non-AIDS Patients
Toxoplasma gondii	*Cryptococcus*
Cytomegalovirus	*neoformans*
Cryptococcus	*Listeria monocytogenes*
neoformans	*Aspergillus fumigatus*
Mycobacterium	*Pseudomonas aeruginosa*
tuberculosis	*Hemophilus influenzae*
Papovavirus (PML)	Klebsiella
Herpes simplex 1 and 2	Varicella zoster
Candida albicans	*Herpes simplex* I
Mycobacterium avium	Enterovirus
intracellulare	*Nocardia asteroides*
Coccidioidomycosis	*Mycobacterium*
Nocardia asteroides	*tuberculosis*
Treponema pallidum	Mucormycosis
Epstein-Barr virus	*Streptococcus*
Varicella zoster	*pneumoniae*
	Toxoplasma gondii
	Papovavirus (PML)
	Candida albicans
	Strongyloides stercoralis

[a] Arranged roughly in order of relative frequency
with most frequent at top.

epidural abscess, that are outside the nervous system but incidentally impinge on it. Even with infections remote from the nervous system, metabolic complications may produce neurologic signs and symptoms. With *Pneumocystis carinii* pneumonia, severe hypoxia may produce obtundation; with *Isospora belli* enteritis, malabsorption may produce peripheral neuropathies.[13] Neither *Pneumocystis* nor *Isospora* organisms cause infections in the nervous system, yet both affect nervous system function.

Multiple organisms may infect the immunodeficient patient simultaneously[1,7,14,15] (Table 4-2). *Pneumocystis car-*

inii pneumonia, oral candidiasis, and toxoplasma encephalitis commonly develop concurrently.[7] Several problems may even occur inside the nervous system simultaneously, but more typically the AIDS patient has a neurologic disease concurrently with several systemic infections. Patients with subacute encephalitis from the human immunodeficiency virus also have *Pneumocystis carinii* pneumonia or systemic cytomegalovirus infection or both in two out of three cases.[16] One patient with a nocardial brain abscess concurrently exhibited oral candidiasis, cytomegalovirus retinitis, and pulmonary nontuberculous mycobacteriosis.[17] Oral candidiasis has been reported in over 40 percent of patients with HIV subacute encephalitis.[16] Perianal herpes simplex or metastatic Kaposi's sarcoma develops in about one-third of those with subacute encephalitis.[16]

Individual organ systems may be attacked at the same time by two or three organisms. Cytomegalovirus and herpes simplex may simultaneously infect the central nervous system of the patient with AIDS.[14] Nonviral infections responsible for much of the mortality seen with AIDS are from *Toxoplasma gondii, Cryptococcus neoformans, Candida albicans,* and *Mycobacterium* species.[1,3,17] Distinguishing among these different infections when they affect the central nervous system requires serologic and CSF measurements and identification of organisms in culture. Neuroimaging techniques are usually helpful in diagnosis but are rarely sufficient. Most opportunistic infections require cerebrospi-

Table 4-2. Common Opportunistic Infections in AIDS Patients

Class of Agent	Primarily Systemic	Primarily CNS
Protozoa	*Pneumocystis carinii*	*Toxoplasma gondii*
Fungi	*Candida albicans*	*Cryptococcus neoformans*
		Coccidioidomycosis
Bacteria	*Mycobacterium tuberculosis*	*M. avium* intracellulare
	Isospora belli	*Nocardia asteroides*
Viruses	Varicella zoster	Cytomegalovirus
	Epstein-Barr	Papovaviruses
		Herpes simplex

nal fluid studies and brain biopsy for definitive diagnosis.

TOXOPLASMOSIS

Perhaps 25 percent to 50 percent of healthy adults in the United States carry the protozoan *Toxoplasma gondii* asymptomatically.[18,19] Immunocompetent individuals routinely control the spread of the organism through the actions of T lymphocytes and activated macrophages.[20] When infestation produces symptoms, they are usually limited to fever, malaise, and lymphadenopathy unless the patient has a disabled immune system. Before the AIDS epidemic most of the patients with more fulminant disease resulting from this organism had collagen vascular disease, lymphomas, leukemias, or iatrogenic immunosuppression.[2,19,21–24] Since the appearance of AIDS, toxoplasmosis of the central nervous system, as well as of the heart, lung, prostate, and other organs, has become exceedingly common. Toxoplasma granulomas and abscesses are the most common causes of focal brain lesions in patients with AIDS[1] (Table 4-3).

Patients with AIDS who carried asymptomatic *T. gondii* infestations before acquiring their immunodeficiency have an approximately one in three chance of developing cerebral toxoplasmosis at some time during the course of their immune disorder.[1] When neurologic disease does develop with *T. gondii,* it causes a diffuse en-

Table 4-3. Focal Brain Lesions Found at Autopsy

Lesion	Percent of AIDS Victims
Toxoplasma abscesses	13
Primary brain lymphomas	6
Fungal abscesses	3
Progressive multifocal leukoencephalopathy	2

Based on data in Navia et al.[1]

cephalopathy, a meningoencephalitis, or multiple brain abscesses.[1,7,15,19] *T. gondii* abscesses appear in the brains of about 13 percent of AIDS victims who come to autopsy.[1,25] Masses appearing in the brains of AIDS victims from Haiti are even more likely to represent *Toxoplasma* abscesses because the organism is more endemic in Haiti than it is in the United States[1] (Fig. 4-1).

Disease develops in the central nervous system with this organism because of a defect most specifically in cell-mediated immunity.[7,19] *T. gondii* is an obligate intracellular parasite; it cannot survive independent of host cells. Intracellular infections are managed in part by components of the immune system that are destroyed in AIDS, the T lymphocytes. Protozoans not obliged to reside intracellularly are not as likely to flourish in patients with AIDS precisely because elements of the immune system that are more specifically directed against them are spared. During its complex life cycle, *T. gondii* assumes several different mature and immature forms. The stage of the cycle most commonly found in the brain of symptomatic individuals is the trophozoite stage.

Of those patients who present with neurologic problems as the initial indication of AIDS, the overwhelming majority have *Toxoplasma* encephalitis.[1,3] Even when central nervous system toxoplasmosis does not cause the initial overt signs of AIDS, it usually evolves early in the course of the immune disorder, if it is going to occur at all. CNS toxoplasmosis develops weeks or months after the initial manifestations of AIDS, if it is not responsible for the initial signs and symptoms of AIDS.[1,25,26]

Case History One

A 53-year-old woman was admitted to the hospital in 1983 because of headache, agitation, paraparesis, and visual hallucina-

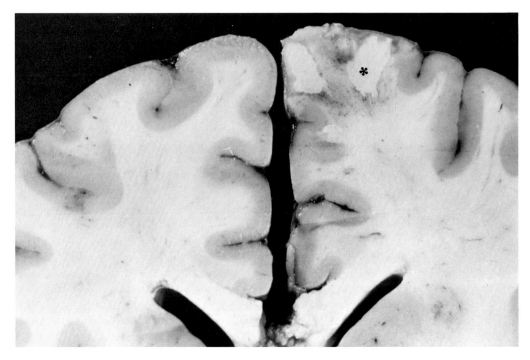

Fig. 4-1. Closeup view of the frontal lobes in coronal section with a *Toxoplasma gondii* granuloma (*) in the right superior frontal gyrus.

tions. Three years earlier she had had a breast resection for the management of breast cancer. During that operation, she received 2 units of blood. Bone marrow metastases were treated with cyclophosphamide, methotrexate, 5-fluorouracil, and tamoxifen. No further metastases became evident, and the patient was continued on tamoxifen until 6 months before this admission.

Three months before the current admission she developed dyspnea, anorexia, and fever. She had an 18 pound weight loss over the preceding few months. Transbronchial biopsy revealed *Pneumocystis carinii* pneumonia. This responded to trimethoprim and sulfamethoxazole (Bactrim), but the patient subsequently developed herpes simplex lesions on her lips and candidiasis of her esophagus. Her immunologic evaluation established a defect in T-lymphocyte function diagnostic of AIDS.

At the time of the final admission, her examination revealed paraparesis. Her cerebrospinal fluid was largely normal except for a slightly elevated protein content (60 mg/dL). Within a few days of hospitalization, the patient became obtunded. The initial computed tomogram of the head revealed no structural lesions. The patient developed an acute pancreatitis. Within a day she had recurrent right focal motor seizures. These were treated with phenytoin and phenobarbital. The adult respiratory distress syndrome developed and treatment with broad spectrum antibiotics was instituted.

A repeat spinal tap revealed no cells, a normal sugar content, and a slight (118 mg/dL) elevation of the protein content. Because of concern that the patient might have a herpes encephalitis, she was started on Ara-A, but she died within 1 day of the initiation of treatment.

At autopsy, this woman had a necrotizing toxoplasma granuloma in her left temporal lobe, which appeared to be in the white matter (Fig. 4-2). On microscopic examination, it had a necrotic center, surrounded by an infiltrate of polymorphonuclear leukocytes and mononuclear cells, as well as macrophages. Small arteries about the granuloloma had fibrous thickening of their walls. Numerous cysts filled with toxoplasma trophozoites were evident in the inflammatory exudate.

This patient probably acquired AIDS while receiving blood transfusions for her cancer surgery. The surgery was done in New York City before blood could be tested for HIV antibodies. As in most cases of AIDS, the initial signs and symptoms were caused by *Pneumocystis carinii* pneumonia, even though she probably had developing central nervous system toxoplasmosis. Computed tomography failed to reveal cerebral toxoplasmosis in this patient even though it was adequately advanced to have a lethal outcome shortly thereafter. Her spinal fluid composition was abnormal, but the abnormalities did not point toward the eventually lethal problem. As is often true in patients with AIDS, there was a progressive acceleration of the clinical deterioration as the disease evolved.

Signs and Symptoms

Clinical signs and symptoms of central nervous system toxoplasmosis are extremely variable. Patients may present with altered mentation, depressed consciousness, seizures, cranial nerve dysfunctions,

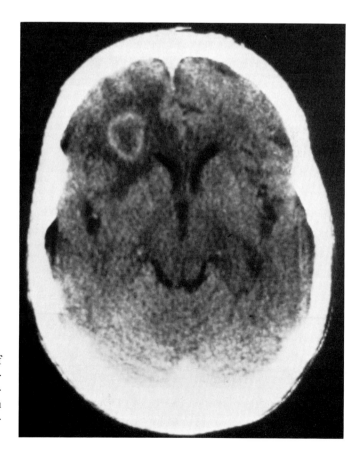

Fig. 4-2. Computed tomogram of toxoplasma granuloma. The ring-enhancing lesion in the right frontal lobe is necrotic tissue with surrounding vascular proliferation and edema.

Table 4-4. Presenting Signs and Symptoms of CNS Toxoplasmosis with AIDS

Focal	Nonfocal	Systemic
Hemiparesis	Headache	Fever
Ataxia	Confusion	
Seizures	Lethargy	
Aphasia	Coma	
Cranial nerve	Behavior disorders	
palsies	Psychomotor	
Dysmetria	retardation	
Movement		
disorders		

focal weakness, or limb spasticity[1,7,27] (Table 4-4). Headache, disorientation, seizures, and hemiparesis are the most common presenting problems.[1,27] Focal signs are more likely when the patient has strictly neurologic damage from the infection (Fig. 4-3). Depressed consciousness and seizures are more typical when the patient has systemic disease along with the central nervous system disease.[7] Cranial nerve palsies occasionally develop and movement disorders, such as chorea, are relatively rare.[1,28] Intracerebral lesions often cause the syndrome of inappropriate secretion of antidiuretic hormone.[7]

In cases with multiple neurologic signs or symptoms, a diffuse encephalopathy is usually the dominant problem.[1] This is characterized by confusion, disorientation, and lethargy. Progressive obtundation is likely with this encephalopathy, and it may be preceded by paranoid delusions, agitation, or anxiety.[1,25,26] Visual hallucinations and delirium may be prominent as the encephalopathy evolves. None of these signs or symptoms of encephalopathy is pathognomonic for toxoplasmic encephalitis.

Most patients with toxoplasmosis have a persistent fever and headache. However, neck stiffness and other signs of meningeal irritation are notably absent in many AIDS patients with CNS toxoplasmosis.[1] Progressive visual loss is occasionally a problem, but this may be from retinal damage caused by either a toxoplasmal or cytomegaloviral chorioretinitis. In patients with prominent dementia and cerebral toxoplasmosis, it is impossible to establish on clinical grounds whether the dementia is from *T. gondii* infection or human immunodeficiency virus injury to the brain.[1]

Diagnosis

Computed tomography of the brain is especially valuable in the assessment of AIDS patients thought to have central nervous system toxoplasmosis.[26,27,29] The computed tomogram done at the time of initial evaluation often reveals an intracranial lesion that eventually establishes the diagnosis.[27] The patient with significant infection will usually exhibit contrast enhancing rings or nodules produced by toxoplasma granulomas.[30] There is often more than one ring or nodule, generally occurring in the white matter, corticomedullary junction, or basal ganglia.[7,31]

The frontoparietal areas are favored sites for *Toxoplasma* granulomas, and three out of four lesions identifiable on computed tomography will be in one of the cerebral hemispheres.[1] These lesions are avascular and are often surrounded by areas of low density.[31] Calcifications are occasionally evident in or about the lesions. Double dose contrast injection may improve the yield of computed tomography, but there are still many more lesions evident when the brain is examined at autopsy than are apparent on computed tomography.[1] Lesions not evident on computed tomography are occasionally apparent with magnetic resonance imaging (MRI).[1]

Establishing that the focal lesion seen on computed tomography or MRI is a *Toxoplasma* granuloma is difficult without performing a brain biopsy. The cerebrospinal fluid may have an elevated protein content, but whether or not glucose levels are depressed or pleocytosis is evident is quite variable.[1] Sabin-Feldman dye tests may yield elevated (more than 1:100) titers in

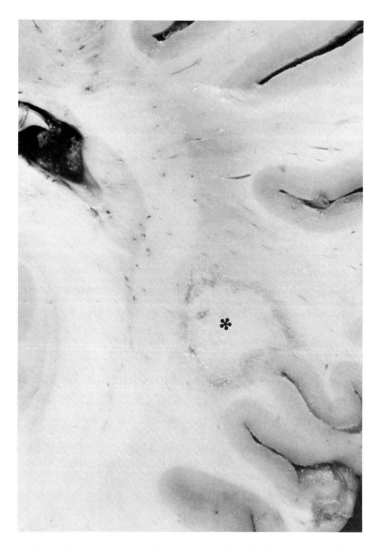

Fig. 4-3. Closeup view of a horizontal section of the optic radiation and occipital lobe white matter with toxoplasma granuloma adjacent to the optic radiation (*). This patient had a visual field defect.

both serum and cerebrospinal fluid, but false-negative results are common with AIDS.[2,7,32] Enzyme-linked immunoabsorbent assay for *Toxoplasma gondii* antibody is useful for detecting evidence of active infection in both the serum and the CSF, and immunofluorescent antibody tests may also be useful, but all of these tests are limited in their usefulness because of the defective immune status of the AIDS patient.[2,7,33] The AIDS patient's antibody response to toxoplasmosis is usually defective.[17]

IgG measured on immunofluorescent antibody tests may be elevated enormously in the AIDS patient infected with *Toxoplasmosa* organisms, but antibody levels may be nonspecifically elevated in AIDS and a generalized hypergammaglobulinemia may mask the IgG elevation. IgG antibody titers against *T. gondii* in the blood are often greater than 1:1,024 when active infection is present.[1,30,34] Low titers in the immunosuppressed patient do not exclude toxoplasmosis but are less common with active infection than are markedly elevated titers.[1,30] Serum and CSF assays for antitoxoplasma IgM are inadequate because they lack specificity and sensitivity.[17] Serum IgM toxoplasma titers are often negative even when the patient has biopsy proven disease.[30] Patients in a population that does not usually exhibit elevated toxoplasma titers, such as Haitians, should be suspected of having toxoplasma encephalitis if they have neurologic signs and a single elevated toxoplasma titer.[30]

Brain biopsy will establish whether or not brain lesions are from toxoplasmosis, but this is a relatively traumatic procedure.[19] If biopsy is needed to establish the diagnosis, it should be performed stereotactically under computed tomographic guidance.[19] Some clinicians believe that the response to therapy is adequately rapid to justify a therapeutic trial before biopsy if evidence suggests that the patient has cerebral toxoplasmosis.[1]

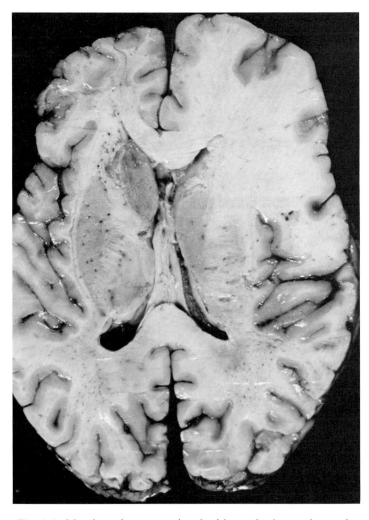

Fig. 4-4. Massive edema associated with cerebral toxoplasmosis.

Histopathology

Grossly, the brain lesion often has a necrotic center surrounded by granulomatous tissue and edema[15] (Fig. 4-4). This granulomatous tissue is composed of acute and chronic inflammatory cells, reactive astrocytes, and macrophages.[1,7] The ring of enhancement evident on contrast-enhanced computed tomography is produced by vascular proliferation around the margins of the granuloma. Marked endothelial hyperplasia usually occurs in these proliferating vessels.[1]

The organism can be cultured from infected biopsy specimens, but this is usually unnecessary.[19] Histologic studies routinely suffice to unequivocally identify the organism. Round or oval organisms, generally in groups, are distributed throughout the inflammatory tissue.[15] The organisms seen are the trophozoite form of the protozoan,[7] an obligate intracellular parasite, which causes cell death upon invasion of cells.[1]

On routine hematoxylin and eosin or Giemsa staining, the responsible organism usually will be evident.[15,19] The organisms are basophilic and occur either free or in pseudocysts around necrotic areas in the brain.[7] The injured brain tissue exhibits vasculitis and infiltrates of large lymphocytes, as well as polymorphonuclear and plasma cells.[7] Lipid-laden macrophages appear in areas with necrotic material.[1]

Most distinctive in the biopsy specimen of many individuals with AIDS is the relative paucity of cellular inflammation in regions with toxoplasma pseudocysts. Perivascular inflammation may be evident at the edge of the toxoplasma granuloma (Fig. 4-5). Because granulomas do not necessarily form and the organisms need not occur in

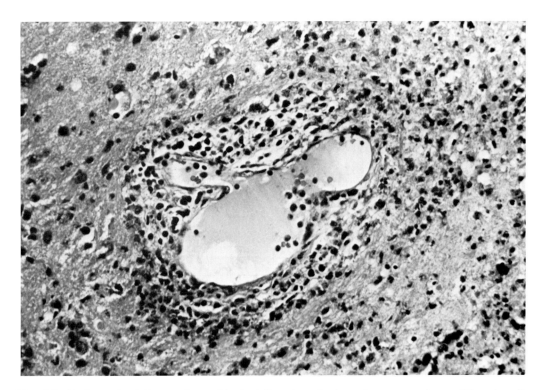

Fig. 4-5. Perivascular inflammation evident at the edge of a toxoplasma granuloma. (Hematoxylin and eosin stain, original magnification ×250.)

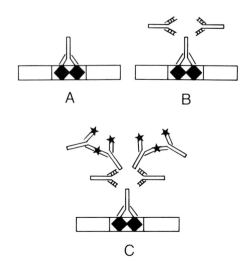

A   B

C

Fig. 4-6. Schematic of peroxidase-antiperoxidase staining technique. An antibody to the toxoplasma which can be linked to a color reaction is incubated with the section. Linking the antibody that binds to organisms in the slide to a color reaction reveals otherwise unsuspected sites where the organism occurs.

clusters, microscopic evidence of infection may be difficult to find. In questionable cases, more specific staining techniques, such as peroxidase-antiperoxidase stains, are available for establishing the diagnosis[1,34,35] (Fig. 4-6).

This staining technique uses antitoxoplasma antibodies linked in various ways to peroxidase enzymes. Isolated organisms can be selectively stained with this technique because the antibodies will attach to material that is otherwise unrecognizable as toxoplasma-derived. Addition of the enzyme substrate produces a color reaction that provides contrast in areas that are linked with the toxoplasma antibodies. (Plate 4-1).

Electron microscopy may reveal the characteristic cysts with protozoa[15] (Fig. 4-7). Toxoplasma organisms are 3 to 7 μm across, crescent-shaped, and aggregated into cysts with five or more protozoans.[15] They occur in the brain in truly cystic and pseudocystic forms. The true cyst has a double membrane; the pseudocyst has a single membrane about the organisms[15] (Fig. 4-8). The pseudocyst is actually a greatly distended cell filled with toxoplasma organisms (Plate 4-2). This infected cell is presumed to be a macrophage.

Treatment

Although the risk of CNS toxoplasmosis is high in certain groups, such as Haitians with AIDS and neurologic signs, many physicians believe that it is wisest to biopsy any brain mass evident in an AIDS patient before initiating treatment[36,37] (Fig. 4-9). Ring-enhancing lesions on the computed tomogram (CT) and positive serologic tests for toxoplasmosis in a patient with AIDS are accepted by other physicians as adequate grounds for initiating therapy without a biopsy.[1,19,31] If ring-enhancing lesions apparent on CT or MRI are not surgically accessible, a therapeutic trial with pyrimethamine and sulfadiazine is certainly reasonable. Nonsurgical intervention is further justified if an initial IgG level indicates no Toxoplasma involvement before the appearance of neurologic signs and a subsequent check reveals a 16-fold or greater increase in Toxoplasma IgG titers.[30] This approach is especially feasible if neurologic signs are not substantial or rapidly progressive.[30] Patients who have already been biopsied for other brain lesions may be better served by a trial of anti-Toxoplasma medications rather than repeated neurosurgical procedures. A response to treatment should be evident symptomatically and on follow-up CT or MRI scan within 2 to 4 weeks of initiating therapy.[30]

Pyramethamine and sulfadiazine are the drugs of choice in the management of central nervous system *T. gondii*.[2,19] They are always used in combination but often produce significant side effects. Sixty percent of AIDS patients treated in this way for toxoplasma encephalitis develop leukopenia,

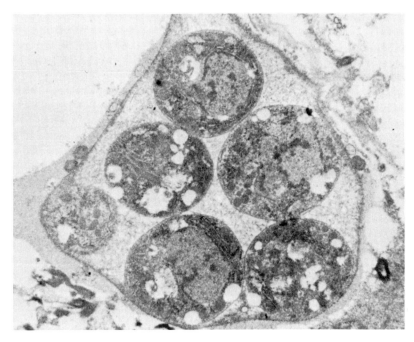

Fig. 4-7. Electron micrograph of six toxoplasma trophozoites in a pseudocyst magnified ×3500.

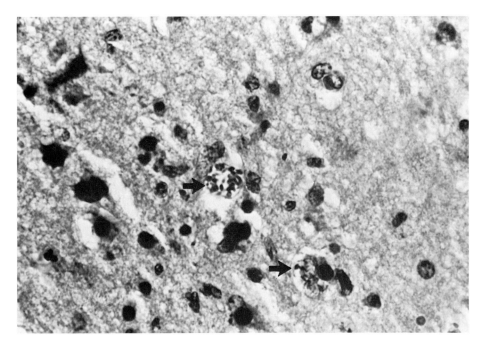

Fig. 4-8. Toxoplasma pseudocyst. This microscopic section shows an inflammatory lesion in the cerebral white matter with pseudocysts (arrows) containing toxoplasma organisms. (Hematoxylin and eosin stain, original magnification ×400.

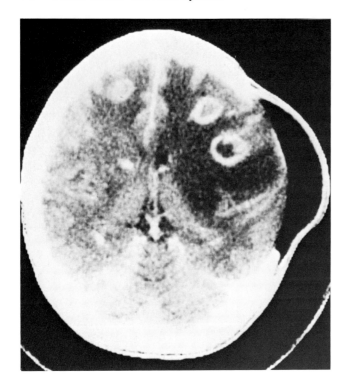

Fig. 4-9. Computed tomogram of toxoplasmosis lesions after biopsy. Multiple ring-enhancing lesions and massive edema are evident.

rash, thrombocytopenia, or other problems that limit the continued use of the drugs.[27] If the patient is allergic to sulfa drugs, intravenous clindamycin may be used instead of sulfadiazine.[1] If cerebral edema is prominent or herniation is impending, dexamethasone may be used transiently.[1]

The elevation of antibody titers and the number of distinct lesions evident in the brain of the AIDS patient with toxoplasmosis do not correlate with the patient's susceptibility to drug treatment.[1,25,26] That multiple abscesses are identifiable on both sides of the brain does not worsen the prognosis. In fact, even the patient's level of consciousness and cerebrospinal fluid abnormalities at the initiation of treatment do not affect the outcome of treatment.[1] All patients with *T. gondii* infection of the central nervous system should be treated vigorously.

How long patients with CNS toxoplasmosis and AIDS must be treated with these drugs is unknown. Some patients have been continued on pyramethamine and sulfonamides for more than 11 months.[1] Rapid improvement does occur in many of the patients treated, with substantial reduction of signs and symptoms occurring within 1 to 2 weeks in the most rapidly responding cases.[1,27] Clearing of the CT or MRI scan does not mean that the patient does not still harbor potentially lethal CNS toxoplasmosis, so these neurodiagnostic modalities cannot be used to determine when therapy should be stopped.[19]

Regardless of treatment, the survival of AIDS patients with toxoplasma encephalitis has been abysmal.[1,7,26,27,29] Median survival from the initiation of treatment has been 126 days, with most patients succumbing within 1 to 18 months after treatment has begun.[7,27] Even with highly effective treatment, the relapse rate is about 30 percent.[8] The use of zidovudine (AZT) may improve longevity, but this has not yet been documented. In any AIDS patient, the possibility of concurrent infection with another opportunistic organism or even concurrent lymphoma must be considered and sought.[1] Concurrent diseases must be treated aggressively if the patient is to survive the CNS toxoplasmosis.

CYTOMEGALOVIRUS

Cytomegalovirus (CMV) is a DNA virus in the herpesvirus group that occurs asymptomatically in most immunocompetent individuals.[12,38] Decades before AIDS first appeared, it was described as causing encephalitis and a variety of systemic diseases in immunodeficient hosts.[4,14,38,39] In the United States, 60 percent to 80 percent of all adults carry the virus and about 1 percent of all live-born infants have evidence of the virus at birth.[11] Prenatal CMV infection can cause extensive nervous system damage in the fetus, but viral acquisition by immunocompetent individuals after birth rarely produces significant illness.[11] In patients with AIDS, the virus may cause widespread damage in the lungs, kidneys, eyes, brain, and other organs. Cytomegalovirus does not exhibit neurotropism, that is, a predilection to infect nervous system tissue, despite its apparent ability to cause extensive nervous system damage in the AIDS patient.[4,14]

Seventy-five percent of patients with AIDS have cytomegalovirus (CMV) infections somewhere in their bodies; these infections routinely produce fever, leukopenia, and pneumonia, as well as damage to the brain.[14] At least 26 percent of patients who die with AIDS have an apparent cytomegalovirus encephalitis, but it is not usually the immediate cause of death.[40,41] Rather, systemic sepsis or overwhelming pneumonia is more likely to kill the patient.[42,43]

Cytomegalovirus is transmitted from human to human—it is species specific.[4,11] The virus can be recovered from saliva, tears, blood, urine, feces, semen, breast milk, and cervical secretions.[11] During pregnancy, it can cross the placenta and cause fetal damage, but in uneventful gestations it usually spares the fetus. To what extent fetal damage occurring in the children of women with AIDS is attributable to prenatal CMV infection is uncertain. CMV is reactivated more frequently during pregnancies than between pregnancies in all women who are actively reproducing, even if the woman does not have AIDS.[11] Consequently, the risk to the fetus of CMV infection in a woman with AIDS is high.

CMV routinely infects the lungs, liver, heart, joints, intestines, eyes, brain, spinal cord, and meninges in susceptible individuals.[11,14] These lesions in all of these organs are inflammatory. Nervous system problems include a Guillain-Barré syndrome, and, indeed, CMV may yet prove to be a frequent cause of the Guillain-Barré syndrome seen in patients with AIDS.[11,44] In the eye, CMV causes a progressive retinitis.[45] In the brain it infects both neurons and glia.[46] Meningeal disease produces a chronic meningitis.[44]

Diagnosis

The signs and symptoms of CMV infection of the nervous system in the patient with AIDS is largely indistinguishable from that seen with toxoplasmosis, and so the diagnosis cannot be based on the clinical history or the physical examination. Patients may present with evidence of an acute meningitis, including fever, neck stiffness, headache, and photophobia.[4,44] More commonly, this virus produces an encephalitis or meningoencephalitis with cognitive deterioration, seizures, and progressive weakness figuring prominently in the clinical course. In some patients, the virus causes a motor polyradiculopathy or chronic meningitis, manifested as a flaccid quadriparesis, psychosis, and dystonia, but it is difficult to establish whether all of these problems are direct effects of the CMV infection.[44]

The eye disease associated with CMV infection is similar to that occurring in newborns after intrauterine cytomegalovirus infection. A chorioretinitis produces patches of retinal damage with associated scotomas.[47] As the disease progresses, white patches with distinct borders spread centrifugally along blood vessels and can be seen on the retina.[6] The lesions evolve over the course of months and are associated with hemorrhage and retinal necrosis. The hemorrhagic perivascular lesions developing with fulminant infection may lead to blindness.[45] If the acute inflammation abates, the retina is left scarred with patches of depigmentation.[6]

Noninvasive diagnostic tests are not very helpful in establishing the diagnosis of progressive cytomegalovirus infection. Electroencephalographic changes are nonspecific, even if the patient has obvious signs of meningoencephalitis. Generalized slowing and some focal sharp wave activity may be evident, but these findings are compatible with innumerable causes of central nervous system infection. The ring-enhancing lesions on computed tomography so common with cerebral toxoplasmosis do not occur with cerebral CMV infection, but the CT findings with CMV infection are otherwise nonspecific. The predilection of the virus for the ependyma in many cases may produce some increased enhancement about the ventricles on postcontrast computed tomography, but this cannot be considered diagnostic even if it can be resolved with the imaging equipment available. The virus can rarely be isolated from the cerebrospinal fluid of infected individuals and is difficult to culture from the brain.[19,38]

CMV chronic meningitis usually produces a CSF pleocytosis with less than 100 cells/μL.[44] Serum anti-CMV IgG antibody titers may also rise acutely, but the hypergammaglobulinemia of AIDS may obscure this increase if it occurs at all.[44] Complement-fixing antibody to CMV may also test positive in the serum of patients with a cytomegalovirus encephalitis.[44] The most direct method of arriving at the diagnosis of CMV encephalitis is brain biopsy, but acquiring brain tissue from the AIDS patient with CMV infection poses hazards for the neurosurgeon collecting the material, as well as the patient from whom the biopsy is taken. The surgeon must take measures to avoid contamination of the operating room staff with HIV infected materials. The patient may have a stormy course of accelerating central nervous system disease, even if the biopsy specimen is small and acquired with little difficulty.

Histopathology

Biopsy material from the central nervous system of patients with CMV encephalitis will routinely have demyelination, neuronal loss, gliosis, and scattered microglial nodules.[19,48] Microglial nodules are especially prominent in cytomegalovirus infection of the brain and are not substantially different from those seen in HIV encephalopathy.[48,49] Some investigators believe that the distribution of microglial nodules in CMV encephalitis is more restricted than that seen with HIV encephalopathy, but support for this view is still tenuous (Table 4-5). Subpial and subependymal distributions of the microglial nodules are more apparent in CMV infections than in HIV encephalopa-

Table 4-5. Distinguishing CMV from HIV Encephalitis

CMV Encephalitis	HIV Encephalitis
CMV-Cowdry type A inclusions in cells	Multinucleated giant cells
Periventricular and subpial microglial nodules	Perivascular microglial nodules
No vacuolation of myelin	Vacuolation of myelin

thy.[44] What is more distinctive about the microglial nodules of CMV encephalitis is the absence of the multinucleated syncytial cells routinely found in HIV infection and the appearance of cells with inclusion bodies.

Intranuclear inclusions, called Cowdry type A inclusions, are prominent in injured cells[48,49] (Fig. 4-10). Cells with the Cowdry type A inclusions may be found in great number in tissue close to the ventricles, including cells of the choroid plexus.[14,49] Cowdry type A inclusions also have been described in retinal ganglion cells.[44] Inclusion material in the nucleus contains cytomegaloviral DNA, which may be selectively labeled with antibody probes that attach to CMV DNA. Such DNA probes

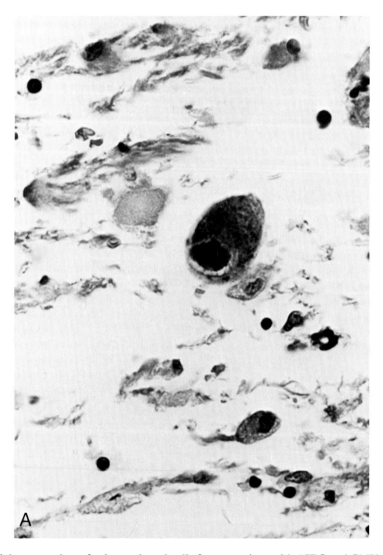

Fig. 4-10. High power view of subependymal cells from a patient with AIDS and CMV ependymitis. **(A)** A dense Cowdry type A inclusion almost fills the nucleus of the cell in the center of the field and inclusion material is also evident in the cytoplasm. (*Figure continues.*)

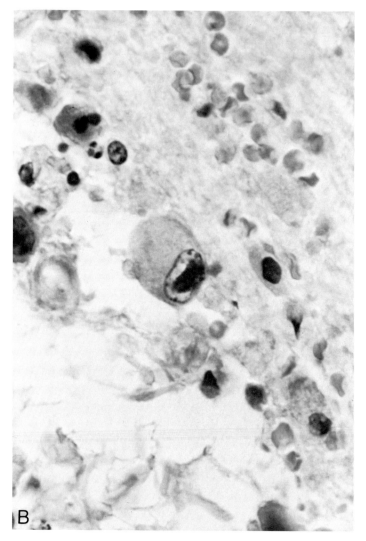

Fig. 4-10. (*continued*) (**B**) The cytomegalic cell, evident in the center of the field, is characteristically larger than cells free of inclusions. (Hematoxylin and eosin stain, original magnification ×400.)

distinguish between intranuclear inclusions produced by CMV and those produced by other viral infections. With CMV infection, inclusion material distinct from the intranuclear body is evident in the cytoplasm of many infected cells.

Throughout the affected brain are areas of demyelination with associated mononuclear inflammatory infiltrates.[4,44] Demyeli- nation may even be found in cranial nerves that are not symptomatic.[44] In subependymal regions numerous cytomegalic cells with Cowdry type A inclusions occur surrounded by microglial cells.[44,48] Some adults with AIDS develop the uncommon form of cytomegalic infection characterized by a necrotizing ventriculitis.[48] Patients with CMV polyradiculopathy have evidence of motor nerve root infection, motor axon destruction, and sparing of the dorsal roots.[44]

Treatment

There is no consistently effective treatment for cytomegalovirus infection of the brain or spinal cord. Cytomegalovirus retinitis has been treated with some success with dihydroxypropoxylmethylguanine.[17] More central disease has been treated with interferon and vidarabine with some reports of improvement.[19] Effective management of cytomegalovirus infection of the central nervous system will probably require suppression of the human immunodeficiency virus.

HERPES SIMPLEX

Herpes simplex is a DNA virus with obvious neurotropism: It can and often does cause an encephalitis or meningitis in immunocompetent, as well as immunodeficient, individuals.[14,50] Most adult cases of herpes encephalitis are caused by herpes simplex type 1.[38] In the immunocompetent patient, this virus produces a hemorrhagic necrotizing encephalitis predominantly affecting the mesial temporal and inferior frontal lobes.[12] This encephalitis is usually an acute, rapidly progressive disease with a mortality rate of 70 percent if no therapy is attempted.[50] Anything less than a fulminant course is distinctly unusual in the immunocompetent patient.[50]

The initial signs of this necrotizing encephalitis include prominent psychiatric phenomena, such as hallucinations and delusions, as well as fever, seizures, obtundation, and aphasia.[51] As the disease evolves, progressive obtundation and seizures are likely.[50] Because of the predilection of herpes virus for the nervous system,

Table 4-6. Characteristics of Herpes Simplex Encephalitis

Immunocompetent Patient	AIDS Patient
Acute or subacute progression	Subacute or chronic progression
Type 1 in adults; Type 2 in neonates	Type 1 or 2 in adults or children
Transient viral antigens in brain	Persistent viral antigens in brain
Hemorrhagic necrotizing lesions	Nonhemorrhagic nonnecrotizing lesions
Focal temporal or frontal lobe damage	Nonfocal damage
Infection by herpes simplex alone	Concurrent CNS infections

herpes simplex type 1 encephalitis is not generally considered an opportunistic infection, but its manifestations in patients with AIDS are adequately distinctive to suggest a unique response to the virus in these immunodeficient patients[8] (Table 4-6).

Herpes encephalitis is more common in adults with AIDS than in the general population, and the virus responsible may be type 1 or type 2.[8,38] These viruses appear to gain access to the central nervous system much more readily in the patient with AIDS than in the patient with intact cellular immunity. Combined infections with cytomegalovirus and herpes simplex virus also have been well documented in patients with AIDS.[48] The course of the encephalitis is much more chronic than acute, and the damage done by the encephalitis is neither focal nor hemorrhagic.

Diagnosis

Evidence of focal temporal edema on MRI or CT associated with signs of a viral meningoencephalitis is highly suggestive of herpes encephalitis in the immunocompetent patient but not usually evident when herpes encephalitis occurs in the patient with AIDS. The periodic lateralizing epileptiform discharges often seen on electroencephalography in the immunocompetent patient with herpetic encephalitis also need not be evident. The cerebrospinal fluid may exhibit a slight depression of the sugar content, elevation of the protein content, and variable levels of pleocytosis, but all of these are too nonspecific to be diagnostic.

The definitive diagnosis of herpes simplex encephalitis in the AIDS patient requires a brain biopsy.[48] Brain tissue may be checked for the presence of virus by using immunofluorescent stains linked to antibodies in serum hyperimmune for both type 1 and type 2 herpes simplex virus.[38] The virus can rarely be isolated from the cerebrospinal fluid of the infected individual.[38]

Pathophysiology

The herpes simplex virus is apparently able to ascend in neural tissue from superficial lesions.[14] Spread to the spinal roots in the sacrum from perianal lesions may explain the high incidence of herpetic ganglioradiculomyelitis and other central nervous system herpetic complications in homosexual men with AIDS.[14] Perianal infection, transmitted by anal intercourse, is probably a common source of the virus in this population at high risk for AIDS. Both type 1 and type 2 virus can cause severe central nervous system disease, such as an ascending myelitis or encephalitis, in the AIDS patient.[14,38]

In immunocompetent victims, the patient has transiently apparent viral antigens in the brain with rapidly evolving hemorrhagic necrosis. With AIDS, the disease appears to follow a more chronic course. The viral antigen persists and hemorrhagic necrosis is not as prominent.[8] Presumably, AIDS alters the immune response to the herpesvirus and makes a herpetic encephalitis less rapidly destructive.[14]

Treatment

Adenine arabinoside or acyclovir may be useful in the management of herpes simplex infections.[50,52,53] Drug treatment must be started early in the course of the disease if it is to be useful. Acyclovir is given as intravenous doses of 10 mg/kg three times daily. A 10-day course is usually required, but the patient's renal function must be considered in determining the final schedule of doses.[54] Adenine arabinoside 15 mg/kg/day has also been given for 10 days as primary treatment for the viral encephalitis.[50] Patients who fail to respond to adenine arabinoside have been treated with acyclovir with some improvement.[38] Type 2 virus may be more responsive to acyclovir, but this has yet to be demonstrated convincingly.[38] Ganciclovir, a nucleoside analogue of guanine, appears to be useful against cytomegalovirus and may even have some efficacy against herpes simplex infection.[55] The principal disadvantage of this drug is its bone marrow toxicity.[48]

FUNGI

Several different fungi cause systemic problems in the AIDS patient, and some directly invade the central nervous system. *Cryptococcus neoformans* is the most common fungus producing central nervous system problems.[56] *Candida albicans* is a much more common cause of fungal infections in AIDS patients overall, but candidiasis is much less likely to extend to the nervous system. The most common neurologic disease attributable to fungal infection in AIDS patients is chronic cryptococcal meningitis or meningoencephalitis. Neurologic problems can also appear as consequences of fungal damage at sites adjacent to the nervous system, such as the myelopathy associated with vertebral infections. Coccidioides often settles in the vertebral body, and blastomyces may produce damage to the pedicles.[57]

Cryptococcus Neoformans

Cryptococcus neoformans is more often responsible for fungal infection of the brain than any other fungus[56] (Fig. 4-11). This is true whether the patient has AIDS, an immunosuppressed state, or largely intact immunity.[2,56] In patients with AIDS it has been found in the central nervous system at autopsy in more than 12 percent of patients, but it is not usually the immediate cause of death.[42,43] Patients with cryptococcal infection routinely have lung and lymph node dissemination of the fungus and die of opportunistic lung infections or sepsis.[42,43,58]

Cryptococcus is generally considered strictly opportunistic, and a defect in cell-mediated immunity is presumed in any individual who develops an infection with this organism, even though some patients who develop cryptococcal meningitis have no demonstrable immunodeficiency. This fungus occurs widespread in the soil, is occasionally disseminated by infected birds, and is most often contracted via the respiratory tract.[59] Cryptococcal meningitis is responsible for the neurologic signs and symptoms in about one out of four patients who have neurologic disease as the initial manifestation of their acquired immunodeficiency.[3] It is much less common than toxoplasmosis

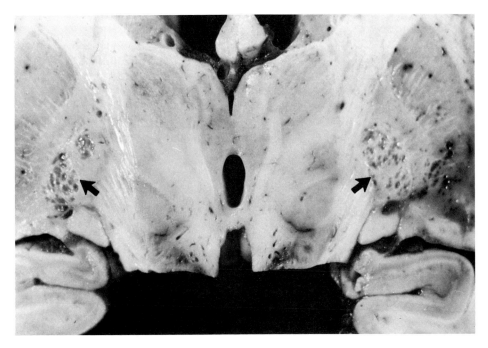

Fig. 4-11. Coronal section through the thalamus and subthalamus in patient with AIDS and cryptococcosis. In the globus pallidus bilaterally there are numerous, small cystic spaces, which represent dilated perivascular spaces filled with cryptococcal organisms (arrows). These are often called soap-bubble lesions because of their gross appearance. The notable reflection of light from the cysts is characteristic of cryptococcal lesions. The capsules of the organisms are mucoid and give the cysts a gelatinous appearance on gross inspection.

of the brain, but it occurs frequently enough to cause problems in diagnosis when the patient does not have the ring-enhancing lesions that suggest toxoplasmic abscess on CT.

Granulomatous meningitis or intracerebral cryptococcomas may develop in patients with AIDS and cryptococcal infections.[8] Early in the evolution of symptoms, the patient may have little more than headache or lethargy.[2,59] Seizures and fever may develop but are not invariably present. Cranial nerve signs, such as diplopia, develop in some patients, but this fungal infection may also present with little more than progressive dementia. Indeed, evidence of disease outside the nervous system may be entirely lacking.[59] Nausea and vomiting may develop if there is increased intracranial pressure. All clinical signs of central nervous system cryptococcal infection are quite variable in the patient with AIDS.

Computed tomography generally does not reveal any focal abnormalities.[31] Examination of the cerebrospinal fluid is much more useful in establishing the diagnosis. The cerebrospinal fluid pressure may be elevated, a lymphocytic pleocytosis may be evident, and the glucose content of the fluid may be slightly depressed.[2] The organism may be evident on India ink preparations but is more often absent.[8] Individuals with AIDS may mount so slight an inflammatory response to central nervous system cryptococcal infection that the cerebrospinal fluid will be normal in all respects except for the presence of cryptococcal antigen or organisms. [8] Latex agglutination tests for cryptococcal antigen are easily performed and usually accurate.[60,61] Cultures for the fungus are falsely negative in more than 10 percent of cases, but cultures of both the cerebrospinal fluid and peripheral blood are appropriate.[2,59,61]

Infected nervous system tissue exhibits remarkably little inflammation.[62,63] Granuloma formation is slight if at all present, even if numerous organisms are evident in and about blood vessels. Biopsy specimens may reveal the organisms in perivascular spaces or in the brain parenchyma itself (Fig. 4-12).

The treatment of choice in all patients with cryptococcal meningitis or cryptococcomas is amphotericin B,[2] which is administered intravenously by daily infusions given over the course of 2 to 6 hours. Amphotericin B is extremely toxic and should only be administered by individuals familiar with adverse reactions. A test dose of 1 mg in 100 cc D5W is usually given before the patient is given a slowly increasing dose not exceeding 0.5 to 0.6 mg/kg. Some physicians use 5-fluorocytosine (5-FC) as well, but the advantages of this medication have not been well established.

Both medications have significant side effects. Amphotericin B is toxic to the kidneys, and 5-FC is toxic to the bone marrow.[2] Some AIDS patients are treated with continuing weekly doses of amphotericin B on an outpatient basis because relapse invariably occurs in this group of patients.[59] Until a successful treatment for AIDS is available, some type of maintenance therapy is needed for the life of the patient. Direct instillation of these drugs into the ventricles by way of an Ommaya reservoir has been advocated by some neurologists, but the survival with cryptococcal meningitis in all patients with AIDS has been poor.[8,56]

Coccidioidomycosis

Coccidioidomycosis is a common fungal infection, which occurs throughout the southwestern United States and affects the lungs primarily. In immunocompetent patients, this fungus may cause a chronic, relapsing meningitis, but in the AIDS patient it is likely to produce a fulminant meningoencephalitis.[8] Treatment has traditionally

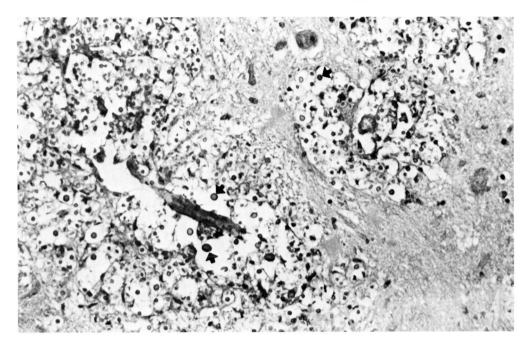

Fig. 4-12. Perivascular areas in the basal ganglia infiltrated by cryptococci. There is virtually no inflammation associated with this dense accumulation of cryptococcal organisms. The clear zones around the darkly staining organisms (arrows) are the capsules of the fungi. (Periodic Acid Schiff stain, original magnification ×250.)

required amphotericin B managed in the same way as required for a cryptococcal meningitis.

Candida Albicans

Candida albicans is a fungus that usually causes superficial infections in immunocompetent patients, but it can be disseminated in the AIDS patient and result in central nervous system infections. *C. albicans* abscesses may develop in the brain,[8,53] which on CT appear to be focal-enhancing lesions.[31] These should be surgically drained and excised. After surgery, treatment includes amphotericin B and 5-FC.[53] Some physicians also use sulfonamides, nystatin, or streptomycin in the management of *C. albicans*.[8]

PROGRESSIVE MULTIFOCAL LEUKOENCEPHALOPATHY

Progressive multifocal leukoencephalopathy (PML) is a demyelinating disease of the central nervous system, which causes focal neurologic signs and cognitive deterioration.[64,65] Signs and symptoms of this disease evolve over the course of weeks or months.[64,66] Without treatment, few patients survive more than 20 months.[66,67] It is caused by CNS infection with a papovavirus and usually occurs only in individuals who have a defect in immunity.[68,19,69] Papovaviruses that usually cause progressive multifocal leukoencephalopathy include the JC and BK viruses, both of which are routinely acquired in childhood.[2,12] At least 70 percent of adults have had an incidental infection with one of the responsible papovaviruses, and yet exceedingly few develop progressive multifocal leu-koencephalopathy.[68] PML is a viral disease of the nervous system, but it is in all respects an opportunistic infection.

Diagnosis

Computed tomography will usually reveal multiple areas of hypodensity in the cerebral white matter, but these nonenhancing lesions are not specific for PML and are indistinguishable from lesions developing with other demyelinating diseases, such as multiple sclerosis, and nondemyelinating diseases, such as CMV encephalitis or HIV subacute encephalitis.[19,70] Other noninvasive studies, including MRI, are equally nonspecific. Unlike with multiple sclerosis, the cerebrospinal fluid does not usually have oligoclonal bands of immunoglobulins.[68] In patients with AIDS, concurrent infections may confuse the picture by eliciting immunoglobulin elevations that are not provoked by the papovavirus.[68]

Most patients have demyelinating lesions scattered throughout the brain[68] (Fig. 4-13). Unlike the demyelination characteristic of multiple sclerosis, however, these lesions evolve simultaneously and show no special affinity for the optic nerves. About 10 percent of patients with PML exhibit lesions predominantly in the brain-stem and cerebellum[68] (Fig. 4-14). It can be diagnosed while the patient is alive only by brain biopsy.[19]

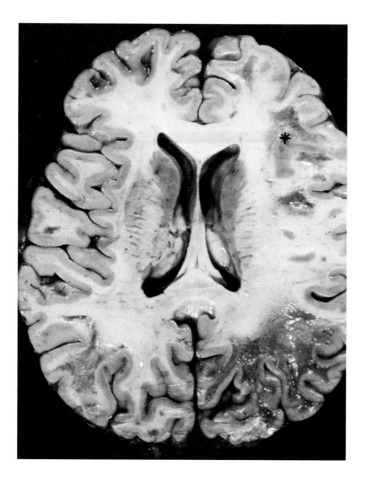

Fig. 4-13. Horizontal section of the brain through the frontal, parietal, and occipital lobes revealing large white matter lesions associated with progressive multifocal leukoencephalopathy. There is discoloration and softening of white matter in the right frontal (*) and both occipital lobes, as well as scattered smaller white matter lesions. These are areas of demyelination in PML.

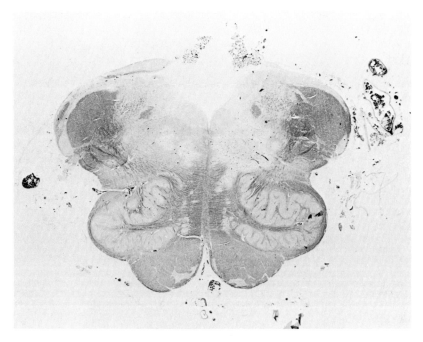

Fig. 4-14. Brain stem demyelination with PML. This section of medulla was stained for myelin and reveals extensive subependymal demyelination caused by PML in the region adjacent to the fourth ventricle. (Myelin stain, original magnification ×3.)

Examination of cells in the cerebrospinal fluid may reveal viral antigen by immunofluorescence.[66] Simian virus 40 (SV40) antigen has been demonstrated in some affected patients by this method.[66] JC virus and BK virus have also been isolated from patients with progressive multifocal leukoencephalopathy.[68] Antibody titers against all of these papovaviruses are not usually high in AIDS patients with progressive multifocal leukoencephalopathy.[68] Presumably, the patient's immunosuppressed state interferes with the antibody reaction.

Histopathology

Brain biopsy will usually reveal extensive areas of demyelination with relative sparing of axons.[68] There are no substantial abnormalities in the gray matter. Phagocytic ac-

tivity is prominent in the white matter and microglial proliferation may be evident[66,68] (Fig. 4-15). Bizarre giant astrocytes may be seen. Oligodendroglial nuclei are swollen and contain large dark-staining inclusions[66] (Fig. 4-16). With electron microscopy, filamentous virions, 33 to 39 nm in diameter, can be seen in these nuclei[68] (Fig. 4-17).

CASE HISTORY

A 29-year-old Hispanic man was admitted to the hospital in 1985 because he was having recurrent episodes of involuntary movements. He had been an intravenous drug abuser for about 5 years, but he claimed to have been drug-free for at least 5 months. The involuntary movements consisted of twitching of his left arm, followed by twisting of the left side of his face and

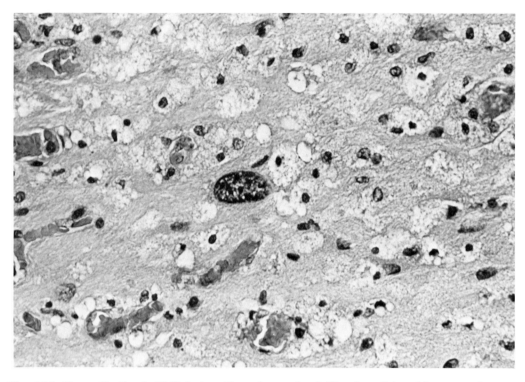

Fig. 4-15. Demyelination in PML lesion. There is massive infiltration of the white matter by macrophages with foamy cytoplasm, reflecting the uptake of lipid from myelin breakdown. The large nucleus in the center of the section is in a giant bizarre astrocyte. (Hematoxylin and eosin stain, original magnification ×250.)

stiffening of his left leg. These lasted 2 minutes and were accompanied by neither premonitory phenomena nor residual weakness. Episodes occurred as often as twice an hour. He had noticed progressive weakness in his left arm and leg, which was independent of the movements and had developed over the course of 3 weeks.

Additional complaints included right occipital headaches, which woke him from sleep, and neck pain, which was worse on awakening. He had night sweats, fever, and cough, associated with foul-smelling sputum and a 40-pound weight loss over the course of 4 months. He also had recently developed hoarseness and difficulty swallowing.

Examination at the time of admission revealed cervical, clavicular, and inguinal lymphadenopathy. Soft rhonchi were apparent posteriorly over the right hemithorax. He was alert, but had a flat affect and poor insight. Tone was increased in the left arm and leg, and strength was slightly impaired, especially in his hand flexors and hip flexors. Sensation was decreased to pain in the left leg. The examination was otherwise unremarkable.

His chest x-ray revealed perihilar infiltrates, but tuberculin skin tests were normal. He did have an obvious leukopenia, with prominent depression of the lymphocyte count. The cerebrospinal fluid was normal except for a slight increase in the protein content (81 mg/dL). Cultures and stains of the cerebrospinal fluid were all negative. Computed tomography of the brain revealed compression of the left ventricle by

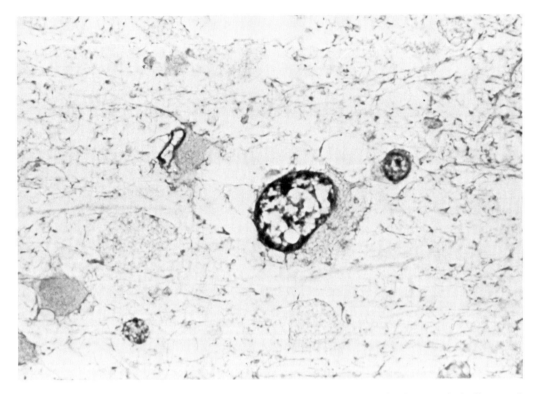

Fig. 4-16. Bizarre giant astrocyte in PML. This type of giant astrocyte is characteristically seen in the cellular reaction in PML. (Hematoxylin and eosin stain, original magnification ×400.)

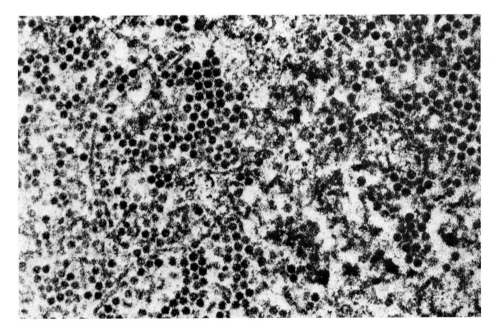

Fig. 4-17. Electron microscopic view of papovavirions from a case of PML. The virus measures 33 to 45 nm across (magnified ×50,000).

a large area of decreased density. The electroencephalogram showed diffuse slowing of the background activity over the right hemisphere, with excessive slowing posteriorly.

The patient was started on anticryptococcal medication empirically but did not improve. A brain biopsy was performed to identify the cause of his left hemiparesis, but he developed aspiration pneumonia shortly after the surgery and died.

The biopsy material had areas of yellowish discoloration evident on gross examination. Microscopic examination revealed multifocal leukoencephalopathy. Macrophages were filled with foamy cytoplasm, acquired from lipid breakdown in the myelin sheaths of nerve fibers (Fig. 4-18). Many oligodendroglial cells had nuclear inclusion bodies. Electron microscopic studies on this tissue revealed intranuclear crystalline arrays of viral particles. Each particle measured 37 to 39 nm across and appeared consistent with papovavirus.

This patient had AIDS complicated by progressive multifocal leukoencephalopathy. Although the patient's initial complaints were probably focal motor seizures, his terminal disease proved to be a strictly white matter lesion. The focal seizures may have been a manifestation of an HIV encephalopathy that was coincidental with the PML. The problems typically encountered in the diagnosis of PML were encountered in this patient and contributed to the misdiagnosis of cryptococcal meningitis. The course of the illness was indistinguishable from a subacute encephalitis secondary to

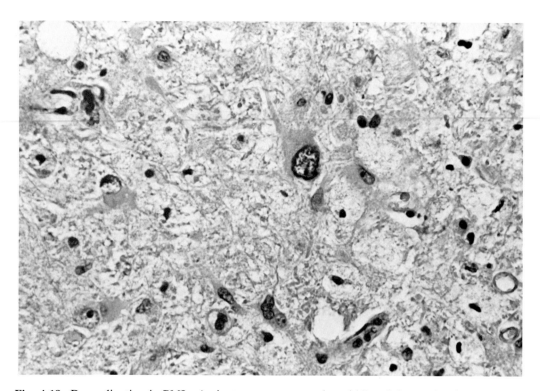

Fig. 4-18. Demyelination in PML. A giant astrocyte near the middle of the section is surrounded by demyelinated white matter. Macrophages with small dense nuclei and foamy cytoplasm are scattered throughout the section. (Hematoxylin and eosin stain, original magnification ×250.)

bacterial or viral disease, and had no features especially suggestive of a demyelinating illness.

CASE HISTORY THREE

A 32-year-old woman with many years of IV cocaine abuse and alcoholism was admitted in 1984 to a psychiatric facility for management of severe depression. Over the 4 months before her admission, she had lost 30 pounds, and this was misconstrued as a vegetative sign of a reactive depression. Shortly after her admission, she had focal motor seizures on the right side of her body. Bilateral myoclonic jerks were also apparent, and a neurologic investigation was begun.

Her examination revealed a right hemiparesis, decreased proprioception on the right, and oral candidiasis. Computed to-mography of the head was unrevealing, and her cerebrospinal fluid was unremarkable, except for oligoclonal bands and a 25 percent IgG component of the total protein.

Seizures became multifocal over the ensuing weeks, and the patient became more lethargic. Her gait was unsteady and broad-based, but she was still adequately intact 3 months after her initial admission to complain of left-sided weakness. The right hemiparesis persisted, and the patient exhibited considerable dysarthria, as well as right hand tremor and bilateral dysmetria. Repeat CT of the brain revealed bilateral white matter hypodensities. She continued to deteriorate and died 5 months after the initial admission for depression.

At autopsy, the patient had AIDS with progressive multifocal leukoencephalopathy. There were numerous irregular lesions in the white matter (Fig. 4-19) characterized by rarified white matter, occasionally with

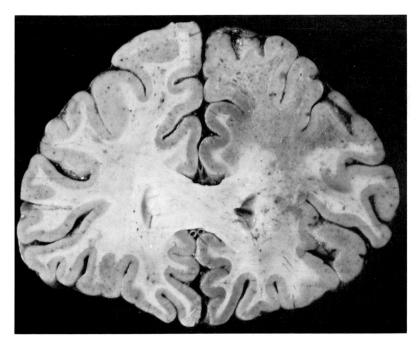

Fig. 4-19. Coronal section through the frontal lobes at the level of the genu of the corpus callosum in PML. A large area of demyelination in the right frontal lobe of the brain is apparent.

cystic degeneration, and numerous glial cells (Fig. 4-20). Most of the glial cells were reactive, but there was also a large population of Alzheimer type II astrocytes and bizarre astrocytes with hyperchromatic nuclei. Lesions in the midbrain exhibited astrocytes with large hyperchromatic nuclei. Some perivascular microglial nodules were evident in the midbrain. Lesions were also found in the medulla and the cerebellum.

No treatment was attempted on this patient because no diagnosis was reached before death. With progressive multifocal leukoencephalopathy, patients are often believed to have a progressive degenerative disease, but the basis for that progressive disease may be obscure. A brain biopsy would have clarified what was causing the deterioration in this patient, but obtaining consent from a depressed or minimally impaired patient may be impossible until the disease is advanced.

Treatment

If biopsy establishes the diagnosis of PML, the physician can justify instituting antiviral therapy.[19,67] Treatment with vidarabine and interferon has produced little improvement.[19]

Cytarabine may be more useful.[19,66,67] It is usually administered at a dose of 60 mg/m^2 intravenously for 6 days and 10 mg/m^2 intrathecally twice.[66] If the patient responds to antiviral therapy, the course of the recovery will usually be as protracted as the course of the deterioration and the recovery is unlikely to be complete (Fig. 4-21). Con-

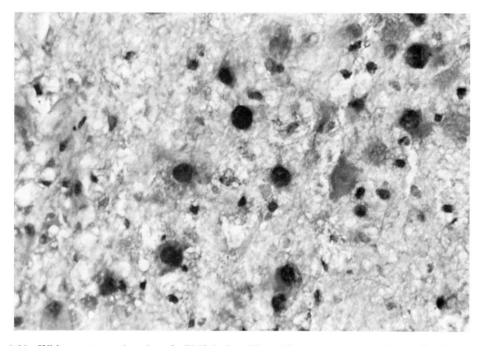

Fig. 4-20. White matter at the edge of a PML lesion. The white matter contains large oligodendroglial nuclei with darkly-staining inclusion material derived from the papovavirus. (Hematoxylin and eosin stain, original magnification ×400.)

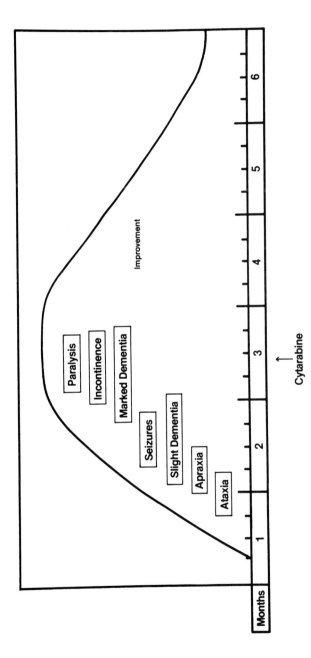

Fig 4-21. Graphic representation of typical time course of neurologic deterioration in PML and the expected rate of recovery if the patient responds to antiviral therapy.

current treatment with zidovudine (AZT) has not yet been described. Most patients with AIDS and PML die within weeks or months, regardless of the treatment instituted.

NOCARDIA

Nocardia asteroides is ubiquitous in the soil, and it is acquired primarily through inhalation.[17] Individuals susceptible to *Nocardia* infection generally have either respiratory disease or impaired immunity.[2] This fungus-like bacterium can thrive in the immunosuppressed host because it impairs phagocytic function in polymorphonuclear cells.[17] Despite the expected vulnerability of the AIDS victim, *N. asteroides* infections account for only 0.3 percent of the infections developing in AIDS patients.[17] The infection arises in the lung and spreads to

the nervous system through the bloodstream in 40 percent of patients infected.[17] The brain is a favored site for extension of the nocardial infection, and brain abscess is the most common manifestation of that infection[2,17] (Fig. 4-22). Multiple foci of infection in the brain are uncommon.[17]

Diagnosis

Initial complaints usually suggest a brain mass but are not specific for nocardial infection. Patients often have fever, headache, and focal neurologic deficits.[2] What sort of focal deficits occur depends on the location of the abscess in the brain. The computed tomogram may exhibit a multiloculated lesion that enhances with contrast.[17] Multiple abscesses or meningitis are much less common than solitary abscesses.[2]

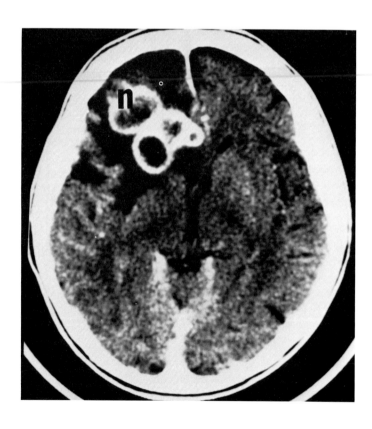

Fig. 4-22. Computed tomogram of nocardial cerebral abscess (n). (From Adair, et al,[12] with permission.)

There may be no sign of nocardial infection outside the CNS, but if there is pulmonary nocardial infection and an abscess consistent with Nocardia organisms, the probability that the organism will be found at the time of brain biopsy is high.[17] Usually, pulmonary or cutaneous nocardiosis precedes cerebral involvement.[17] Some physicians argue that biopsy of a probable nocardial brain abscess is inadvisable when the level of suspicion is very high because of the risk of meningeal contamination.[71] With AIDS, the inevitable uncertainty of diagnosis, because of the risk of multiple infections, makes biopsy essential.[17]

The lesions most likely to be confused with a nocardial abscess are CNS toxoplasmosis, a primary CNS lymphoma, atypical mycobacterial abscess, candidal abscess, and bacterial abscesses.[17] Toxoplasmosis is more than ten times as common as nocardial abscess, so the diagnosis of Nocardia must be supported by more definitive evidence than a suggestive CT scan or MRI.

Treatment

Pulmonary Nocardia is treated with sulfamethoxazole and trimethoprin; these same antibiotics may be useful in managing cerebral Nocardia.[17] If an abscess forms in the brain, it should be drained, preferably stereotactically.[17] Minimal inhibitory concentrations of sulfamethoxazole for the isolate obtained should be checked and the dose of IV medication adjusted accordingly.[17] If leukopenia is substantially exacerbated by these antibiotics, oral sulfadiazine sodium may be used as an alternative, but the urine must be monitored to check for signs of stone formation.[17] Such signs would include hematuria and excessive sulfa crystals. Minocycline HCL has been used as a third line drug.[17]

OTHER INFECTIONS

In any patient with AIDS, there is substantial risk of a conventional meningitis, but this is especially true in infants and children with AIDS. Any evidence of meningitis must be investigated with routine bacterial cultures. Antibiotic coverage will be determined by culture results. Common pathogens found include gram-negative bacteria, such as *Escherichia coli,* and *Treponema pallidum.*[8,10]

Neurosyphilis

Meningovascular syphilis must be routinely sought in patients with HIV infection because the risk of all sexually transmitted diseases is increased in homosexual men with AIDS and the viability of spirochetes in the central nervous system is probably enhanced in all patients with AIDS.[10,72] Indeed, some clinicians consider a history of syphilis as a risk factor for the acquisition of AIDS.[10] This may be too broad a view, but it is undeniable that a history of multiple venereal infections is found in many of the people who develop AIDS.

Patients with primary or secondary syphilis, infections which do not extend to the central nervous system, may develop neurosyphilis, even if they have been treated with routine doses of penicillin, if they have immunodeficiency.[10,72] The effective doses of penicillin widely recommended for syphilitic infections presume that the patient's immune system can make a substantial contribution to the elimination of the infection. Insufficiently treated syphilis in any individual may find its way into the central nervous system. With AIDS, the spirochete seems to find its way into the central nervous system with uncommon ease.[10]

Neurosyphilis is usually diagnosed on the basis of positive VDRL or FTA-ABS tests performed on cerebrospinal fluid. With meningovascular syphilis and AIDS, the cerebrospinal fluid protein is usually elevated slightly and a mononuclear pleocytosis is evident.[10] Brain biopsy is generally not considered necessary, but biopsy material will reveal the spirochete with special silver stains.

The course of neurosyphilis in affected patients is greatly accelerated, another feature suggesting a major impact of the HIV infection.[72] The meningovascular form of neurosyphilis, a problem usually seen 5 to 12 years after syphilis is acquired, may develop within months of a primary infection.[10] General paresis, a progressive degenerative disease caused by spirochetal invasion of brain parenchyma, has yet to be described in patients with AIDS.

Although experience in treating neurosyphilis associated with AIDS has been limited, it is advisable to treat routine syphilitic infections in these patients with regimens that would ordinarily be considered appropriate only for meningovascular syphilis. Intravenous penicillin G administered daily for up to 10 days may be necessary to fully suppress the infection.

Mycobacterium Tuberculosis

Some of the first cases of AIDS described involved Haitians with active tuberculosis.[45] This disease is endemic in Haiti, so its appearance in immunosuppressed individuals was hardly surprising. Although Haitians are no longer considered an extraordinarily high risk group, *Mycobacterium tuberculosis* infection is still commonly associated with AIDS in this group. Tuberculosis infection is an even more prominent component of AIDS in Africa.[73] Patients with pulmonary tuberculosis are at risk of developing tuberculous meningitis in association with disseminated tuberculosis. Conventional antituberculous therapy with isoniazid, rifampin, and ethambutol is effective in patients with tuberculous meningitis.

Mycobacterium Avium Intracellulare

As other patients were evaluated for mycobacterial infections, nontuberculous mycobacteria were found. *Mycobacterium avium intracellulare* is an organism that usually causes disease in chickens and swine but is strictly opportunistic in humans. It occurs with unprecedented frequency in individuals with AIDS and has been cultured from their brains. Even when this organism cannot be recovered from the cerebrospinal fluid, but has been cultured from elsewhere in the body, it may still be present in the brain and cause an encephalopathy.[49] Granulomatous lesions developing as a result of these nontuberculous mycobacteria have not been described.

Clofazimine, a drug used for many years to treat leprosy, has recently demonstrated usefulness against *Mycobacterium avium,* although it has not been officially approved for this use in the United States.[74] This drug is usually given along with more conventional antituberculous drugs, such as ethambutol, rifampin, and isoniazid.[74] The effective doses of these drugs in patients with AIDS are the same as that used in disseminated tuberculosis. Fifty to 100 mg of clofazimine is also administered in some centers.[74]

Epstein-Barr Virus

Epstein-Barr virus also flourishes in patients with AIDS. Some studies suggest that this virus may play a central role in the transformation of lymphocytes into the neoplastic cells found in the non-Hodgkin's lymphomas that are common in the central nervous systems of AIDS victims. No reliable techniques are available to assess the activity of Epstein-Barr virus in AIDS patients, but that will change as more attention is focused on this virus. There is no effective treatment for Epstein-Barr viral infection.

Varicella Zoster

Varicella zoster viruses are herpesviruses that routinely lie dormant in adults after they are acquired and have been symptomatic in childhood. Whether or not varicella zoster is responsible for some of the aseptic meningitides that develop in AIDS patients is controversial. Radicular lesions attributable to reactivated zoster virus certainly do occur, and the patient may have a coincidental aseptic meningitis, but that the meningitis and the radicular lesions are related is difficult to establish.[75] Some patients with varicella zoster virus infections develop myelitis, polyneuritis, or encephalitis apparently caused by or related to nervous system involvement by this herpesvirus.[75]

Tissue from AIDS patients with zoster encephalitis exhibit Cowdry type A intranuclear inclusion bodies and herpes-like nucleocapsids in some cases.[75] Establishing that varicella zoster is the agent responsible for the viral encephalitis is difficult because this herpesvirus is difficult to culture and may be present in material infected by other viruses. Because patients with AIDS are at high risk of having herpes simplex encephalitis with Cowdry bodies and herpes nucleocapsid, establishing the diagnosis of varicella zoster infection in these patients is especially difficult.[75]

The true importance of varicella zoster infections may be as a barometer of HIV activity.[59] As the patient's immunodeficiency advances, *H. zoster* infections may become more symptomatic. Skin lesions in the young person with HIV infection may present no substantial risk to the patient but probably indicates an increased pace of deterioration associated with AIDS.[59] In the few cases of slowly progressive encephalitis directly attributable to varicella zoster infection of nervous system tissue, there has been no effective treatment.

CONCURRENT INFECTIONS

Opportunistic infections are common in AIDS, but concurrent infection in the nervous system with several opportunistic agents at the same time is especially typical of the HIV infected individual. Patients with cerebral toxoplasmosis may have evidence of concurrent CMV lesions in the brain and varicella zoster lesions in the peripheral nerves. Nocardial lesions in the brain do not preclude the appearance of CMV lesions in the brain or the retina. HIV subacute encephalitis can evolve at the same time that the patient's central nervous system is being attacked by herpes simplex or BK papovavirus. As stressed throughout this chapter, this has serious implications for the investigation and treatment of nervous system lesions in AIDS patients. Patients may require therapy for several different infections at the same time.

Drug interactions may pose enormous problems because many of the drugs used against the opportunistic infections developing in the nervous system of AIDS victims have toxic side effects. Some suppress hematopoeisis substantially when given individually and unacceptably when given in combination. An additional consideration in choosing drugs is what effect they will have on agents used against the AIDS virus itself. Antiviral agents effective against progressive multifocal leukoencephalopathy may interfere with the effectiveness of zidovudine (AZT) against HIV. Drugs cannot simply be added as new problems appear. Eventually the cumulative toxicity of the drugs will equal the lethality of the conditions being treated. Any strategy devised to combat opportunistic infections must use drugs with acceptable combined toxicities. The ideal treatment of opportunistic infections developing with AIDS will necessarily start with the elimination or inactivation of the human immunodeficiency virus, a goal which has not yet been achieved.

REFERENCES

1. Navia BA, Petito CK, Gold JWH, et al: Cerebral toxoplasmosis complicating AIDS: clinical and neuropathological findings in 27 patients. Ann Neurol 19:224, 1986
2. Hooper DC, Pruitt AA, Rubin RH: Central nervous system infections in the chronically immunosuppressed. Medicine (Baltimore) 61:166, 1982
3. Berger JR, Moskowitz L, Fischl M, Kelley RE: Neurologic disease as the presenting manifestation of acquired immunodeficiency syndrome. South Med J 80:683, 1987
4. Hawley DA, Schaefer JF, Schulz DM, Muller J: Cytomegalovirus encephalitis in acquired immunodeficiency syndrome. Am J Clin Pathol 80:874, 1983
5. Fauci AS, Macher AM, Longo DL, et al: Acquired immunodeficiency syndrome: epidemiologic, clinical, immunologic, and therapeutic considerations. Ann Intern Med 100:92, 1984
6. CDC: Revision of the CDC surveillance case definition for acquired immunodeficiency syndrome. MMWR 36:3s, 1987
7. Farkash AE, Maccabee PJ, Sher JA, et al: CNS toxoplasmosis in acquired immune deficiency syndrome: a clinical-pathological-radiological review of 12 cases. J Neurol Neurosurg Psychiatr 49:744, 1986
8. Levy RM, Bredesen DE, Rosenblum ML: Neurologic manifestations of the acquired immunodeficiency syndrome (AIDS): experience at the University of California at San Francisco and review of the literature. J Neurosurg 62:475, 1985
9. Moskowitz LB, Kory P, Chan JC, et al: Unusual causes of death in Haitians residing in Miami: high prevalence of opportunistic infections. JAMA 250:1187, 1983
10. Johns DR, Tierney M, Felsenstein D: Alterations in the natural history of neurosyphilis by concurrent infection with the human immunodeficiency virus. N Engl J Med 316:1569, 1987
11. Bale JF Jr: Human cytomegalovirus infection and disorders of the nervous system. Arch Neurol 41:310, 1984
12. Johnson RT: Viral Infections of the Nervous System. Raven Press, New York, 1982
13. Ros E, Fueyo J, Llach J, et al: *Isospora belli* infection in patients with AIDS in Catalunya, Spain. N Engl J Med 317:246, 1987
14. Tucker T, Dix RD, Katzen C, et al: Cytomegalovirus and Herpes simplex virus ascending myelitis in a patient with acquired immune deficiency syndrome. Ann Neurol 18:74, 1985
15. Vilaseca J, Arnau JM, Bacardi R, et al: Kaposi's sarcoma and *Toxoplasma gondii* brain abscess in a Spanish homosexual. Lancet 1:572, 1982
16. de la Monte SM, Ho DD, Schooley RT, et al: Subacute encephalomyelitis of AIDS and its relation to HTLV-III infection. Neurology 37:562, 1987
17. Adair JC, Beck AC, Apfelbaum RI, Baringer R: Nocardia cerebral abscess in the acquired immunodeficiency syndrome. Arch Neurol 44:548, 1987
18. Krick JA, Remington JS: Toxoplasmosis in the adult—an overview. N Engl J Med 298:550, 1978
19. Snow RB, Lavyne MH: Intracranial space-occupying lesions in acquired immunodeficiency syndrome patients. Neurosurgery 16:148, 1985
20. Johnson WD: Chronological development of cellular immunity in human toxoplasmosis. Infect Immun 33:948, 1981
21. Carey RM, Kimball AC, Armstrong D, Lieberman PH: Toxoplasmosis—clinical experiences in a cancer hospital. Am J Med 54:30, 1973
22. Hakes TB, Armstrong D: Toxoplasmosis—problems in diagnosis and treatment. Cancer 52:1535, 1983
23. Ruskin J, Remington JS: Toxoplasmosis in the compromised host. Ann Intern Med 84:193, 1976
24. Ryning FW, Mills J: *Pneumocystis carinii, Toxoplasma gondii,* cytomegalovirus and the compromised host. West J Med 130:18, 1979
25. Wang B, Gold JWM, Brown AE, et al: Central-nervous-system toxoplasmosis in homosexual men and parenteral drug abusers. Ann Int Med 100:36, 1984

26. Luft BJ, Brooks RG, Conley FK, et al: Toxoplasma encephalitis in patients with acquired immune deficiency syndrome. JAMA 252:913, 1984

27. The T E Study Group: Assessment of therapy for Toxoplasma encephalitis. Am J Med 82:907, 1987

28. Nath JA, Jancovic J, Pettigrew LC: Movement disorders and AIDS. Neurology 37:37, 1987

29. Alonso R, Heiman-Patterson T, Mancall EL: Cerebral toxoplasmosis in acquired immune deficiency syndrome. Arch Neurol 41:321, 1984

30. Pitchenik AE, Fischl MA, Walls KW: Evaluation of cerebral mass lesions in acquired immunodeficiency syndrome. N Engl J Med 308:1099, 1983

31. Elkin CM, Leon E, Grenell SL, Leeds NE: Intracranial lesions in acquired immunodeficiency syndrome. JAMA 253:393, 1985

32. Feldman HA, Lamb GA: A micromodification of the *Toxoplasma* dye test. J Parasitol 52:415, 1966

33. Remington JS, Miller MJ, Brownlee I: IgM antibodies in acute toxoplasmosis: II. Prevalence and significance in acquired cases. J Lab Clin Med 71:855, 1968

34. Hauser WE, Luft BJ, Conley FK, Remington JS: Central-nervous-system toxoplasmosis in homosexual and heterosexual adults. N Engl J Med 307:498, 1982

35. Conley FK, Jenkins KA, Remington JS: *Toxoplasma gondii* infection of the central nervous system. Use of the peroxidase-antiperoxidase method to demonstrate *Toxoplasma* in formalin-fixed paraffin embedded tissue sections. Human Pathol 12:690, 1981

36. Snider WD, Simpson DM, Aronyk KE, Nielsen SL: Primary lymphoma of the nervous system associated with acquired immune-deficiency syndrome. N Engl J Med 308:45, 1983

37. Levy RM, Pons VG, Rosenblum ML: Intracerebral mass lesions in the acquired immunodeficiency syndrome (AIDS). J Neurosurg 61:9, 1984

38. Dix, RD, Bredesen DE, Erlich KS, Mills J: Recovery of herpesvirus from cerebrospinal fluid of immunodeficient homosexual men. Ann Neurol 18:611, 1985

39. Dorfmann LJ: Cytomegalovirus encephalitis in adults. Neurology (NY) 23:123, 1973

40. Koppel BS, Wormser GP, Tuchman AJ, et al: Central nervous system involvement in patients with acquired immunodeficiency syndrome. Acta Neurol Scand 71:337, 1985

41. Anders KH, Steinsapir KD, Iverson DJ, et al: Neuropathologic findings in the acquired immunodeficiency syndrome (AIDS). Clin Neuropathol 5:1, 1986

42. Niedt GW, Schinella RA: Acquired immunodeficiency syndrome: clinicopathologic study of 56 autopsies. Arch Pathol Lab Med 109:727, 1985

43. Moskowitz L, Hensley GT, Chan JC, Adams K: Immediate causes of death in acquired immunodeficiency syndrome. Arch Pathol Lab Med 109:735, 1985

44. Behar R, Wiley C, McCutchan A: Cytomegalovirus polyradiculoneuropathy in acquired immune deficiency syndrome. Neurology 37:557, 1987

45. Vieira J, Frank E, Spira TJ, Landesman SH: Acquired immune deficiency in Haitians. N Engl J Med 308:125, 1983

46. Barnes DM: Brain damage by AIDS under active study. Science 235:1574, 1987

47. Kennedy PGE, Newsome DA, Hess J, et al: Demonstration by in situ hybridization of cytomegalovirus but not human T-lymphotropic virus type III in retinal lesions in patients with the acquired immunodeficiency syndrome. Br Med J 293:162, 1986

48. Laskin OL, Stahl-Bayliss CM, Morgello S: Concomitant Herpes simplex virus type 1 and cytomegalovirus ventriculoencephalitis in acquired immunodeficiency syndrome. Arch Neurol 44:843, 1987

49. Belman AL, Ultmann MH, Horoupian D, et al: Neurological complications in infants and children with acquired immune deficiency syndrome. Ann Neurol 18:560, 1985

50. Sage JI, Weinstein MP, Miller DC: Chronic encephalitis possibly due to herpes simplex virus: two cases. Neurology 35:1470, 1985

51. Lechtenberg R: The Psychiatrist's Guide to Diseases of the Nervous System. John Wiley, New York, 1982

52. Whitley RJ, Soong SJ, Dolin R, et al: Adenine arabinoside therapy of biopsy-proved herpes simplex encephalitis. N Engl J Med 297:289, 1977

53. Levy RM, Pons VG, Rosenblum ML: Intracerebral mass lesions in the acquired im-

munodeficiency syndrome (AIDS). J Neurosurg 61:9, 1984

54. Laskin OL: Acyclovir: pharmacology and clinical experience. Arch Intern Med 144:1241, 1984

55. Laskin OL, Stahl-Bayliss CM, Kalman CM, et al: Treatment with ganciclovir for serious cytomegalovirus infections. J Infect Dis 155:323, 1987

56. Kovacs JA, Kovacs AA, Polis M, et al: Cryptococcosis in the acquired immunodeficiency syndrome. Ann Intern Med 103:533, 1985

57. Rhangos WC, Chick EW: Mycotic infections of bone. South Med J 57:664, 1964

58. Welch K, Finkbeiner W, Alpers CE, et al: Autopsy findings in the acquired immune deficiency syndrome. JAMA 252:1152, 1984

59. Desforges J, Mark EJ: Case record 41-1987. N Engl J Med 317:946, 1987

60. Fisher BD, Armstrong D: Cryptococcal interstitial pneumonia: Value of antigen determination. N Engl J Med 297:1440, 1977

61. Meunier-Carpentier FM, Kiehn TE, Armstrong D: Fungemia in the immunocompromised host: changing patterns, antigenemia, high mortality. Am J Med 71:363, 1981

62. Gal AA, Koss MN, Hawkins J, et al: The pathology of pulmonary cryptococcal infections in the acquired immunodeficiency syndrome. Arch Pathol Lab Med 110:502, 1986

63. Amberson JB, DiCarlo EF, Metroka CE, et al: Diagnostic pathology in the acquired immunodeficiency syndrome: surgical pathology and cytology experience with 67 patients. Arch Pathol Lab Med 109:345, 1985

64. Astrom KE, Mancall EL, Richardson EP Jr: Progressive multifocal leuko-encephalopathy: A hitherto unrecognized complication of chronic lymphatic leukaemia and Hodgkin's disease. Brain 81:93, 1958

65. Richardson EP Jr: Progressive multifocal leukoencephalopathy. N Engl J Med 265:815, 1961

66. Peters ACB, Versteeg J, Bots GTAM, et al: Progressive multifocal leukoencephalopathy. Immunofluorescent demonstration of Simian virus 40 antigen in CSF cells and response to cytarabine therapy. Arch Neurol 37:497, 1980

67. Bauer WR, Turel AP, Johnson KP: Progressive multifocal leukoencephalopathy and Cytarabine. JAMA 226:174, 1973

68. Miller JR, Barrett RE, Britton CB, et al: Progressive multifocal leukoencephalopathy in a male homosexual with T-cell immune deficiency. N Engl J Med 307:1436, 1982

69. Budka H, Shah KV: Papovavirus antigens in paraffin sections of PML brains. Prog Clin Biol Res 105:299, 1983

70. Carroll BA, Lane B, Norman D, Enzmann D: Diagnosis of progressive multifocal leukoencephalopathy by computed tomography. Radiology 122:137, 1977

71. Byrne E, Brophy BP, Perrett LV: Nocardia cerebral abscess: new concepts in diagnosis, management, and prognosis. J Neurol Neurosurg Psychiatry 42:1038, 1979

72. Weiss R: AIDS may affect course of syphilis. Science News 131:391, 1987

73. Kanki PJ, M'Boup S, Ricard D, et al: Human T-lymphotropic virus type 4 and the human immunodeficiency virus in West Africa. Science 236:827, 1987

74. Clofazimine for leprosy and *Mycobacterium avium* complex infections. Med Lett Drugs Ther 29:77, 1987

75. Ryder JW, Croen K, Kleinschmidt-DeMasters K, et al: Progressive encephalitis three months after resolution of cutaneous zoster in a patient with AIDS. Ann Neurol 19:182, 1986

5

Tumors

Uncommon tumors occur with uncommon frequency in patients with AIDS. Although the incidence of lung, breast, rectal, and uterine cancers has not been substantially affected by the AIDS epidemic, the incidence of primary brain lymphomas and metastatic Kaposi's sarcomas greatly exceeds population norms in individuals infected with HIV.[1-3] Central nervous system lymphomas have been described in all groups developing AIDS. Kaposi's sarcoma only rarely metastasizes to the brain or spinal cord. No other tumors have affected the nervous system of the patient with HIV infection as often as these two neoplasms.

PRIMARY LYMPHOMAS

Lymphomas are increased in all immunosuppressed patients, but the incidence of primary central nervous system lymphomas is inordinately high in patients with AIDS.[4-6] This type of lymphoma is distinctly uncommon in patients without AIDS but does occur in some patients with congenital immune deficiency, acquired autoimmune disease, or iatrogenic immunologic disturbances.[7-9] Before the appearance of AIDS, primary central nervous system lymphomas accounted for fewer than 2 percent of the lymphomas diagnosed annually in the United States.[8,10]

Unlike most lymphomas, those associated with AIDS and occurring in the central nervous system often present as intraparenchymal masses, rather than as disseminated tumors.[4,9] Central nervous system lymphomas account for about 5 percent of the neurologic lesions seen in patients with AIDS and are the second most common cause of brain masses in these patients, the most common being toxoplasmosis.[9,11] Lymphomas are more common in adults than children, but they occur in both very young and very old patients with AIDS.

Clinical Manifestations

Patients with central nervous system lymphomas most commonly present with headache, confusion, lethargy, personality changes, and memory loss.[8,9] Focal neurologic signs, such as hemiparesis or ophthalmoplegia, may develop after the appearance of higher cortical function impairments, but many patients never develop focal signs.[8] Some patients remain free of symptoms referable to the lymphoma, whereas others have nervous system complaints that are overshadowed by symptoms caused by systemic disease. As is true in any adult with a brain tumor, seizures may be the first manifestation of the tumor.[9]

Most primary brain lymphomas occur in the frontoparietal region or in the posterior

99

fossa.[8,12] About one-third of the lymphomas will be multifocal at the time they are first recognized.[8] When focal neurologic deficits do appear, they may progress over days or weeks. Once the lymphoma has become symptomatic, a rapid clinical deterioration is routine, rather than exceptional.[8,9] Hemorrhages may develop in primary or metastatic brain lymphomas and cause sudden death.[13] Patients dying from disseminated opportunistic infections or vascular complications of AIDS are occasionally found to have unsuspected brain lymphomas at autopsy.

CASE HISTORY ONE

A 26-year-old woman was admitted to the hospital because of headache that had disabled her for over 1 month. These headaches were pounding in quality, worst in the mornings and evenings, and associated with diplopia for one day before admission. The patient had also noticed drooping of her left eyelid during the day before admission.

She had been well until 4 years before admission, at which time she had an ectopic pregnancy and required a blood transfusion. Two years later she was hospitalized for pneumonia that required 4 weeks of intravenous antibiotic treatment. She had never abused drugs or alcohol, although her husband had used illicit drugs intravenously.

Examination at the time of admission revealed intact intellectual function. She had a fever of 101° F orally. Ptosis, ophthalmoplegia, and left pupillary dilation were consistent with a complete third nerve paralysis. Her neurologic examination was otherwise unremarkable. Laboratory tests revealed a slightly prolonged ESR (60 mm/hr) and a marginally low white blood cell count (3800/μL) with only 10 percent lymphocytes. Computed tomography of the brain and angiography, both carotid and vertebral, were normal. Her cerebrospinal fluid was abnormal with 16 white blood cells/μL, 71 percent of which were polymorphonuclear cells, a protein content elevated to 68 mg/dL, and a glucose depressed to 29 mg/dL.

She was started on penicillin and antituberculous therapy but did not improve. Her cerebrospinal fluid showed persistently abnormal protein, sugar, and cell count values. No malignant cells were found in the cerebrospinal fluid, and all cultures were negative. Her fever persisted and vomiting developed. A positive Babinski sign appeared on the right, but a repeat CT of the brain failed to reveal any focal lesions. Six days after admission, the patient had an acute respiratory arrest and did not recover.

At autopsy she was found to have AIDS with a primary malignant lymphoma of the central nervous system. Tumor cells were distributed widely in the leptomeninges, with concentrations of cells in the hypothalamus, medial temporal lobe, and brain stem areas. Associated with this diffuse infiltration was a necrotizing vasculitis and thrombosis. The immediate cause of death appeared to have been a large hemorrhage into the hypothalamus and brain stem, with extension to the basilar leptomeninges. The third cranial nerve was infiltrated with lymphoma cells bilaterally (Fig. 5-1). There was hemorrhage into both third cranial nerves.

The lymphoma cells were large with scanty cytoplasm and oval or round nuclei. There was relatively little pleomorphism. The large cells had prominent nucleoli. Lymphoma cells were present in the walls of leptomeningeal veins, some of which had fibrinoid necrosis of their walls.

Additional findings included microglial nodules with large macrophages. Several of these nodules had closely associated reactive astrocytosis. In the cerebellum, there were many microglial nodules, some of which were perivascular.

This woman had pathologic findings indicative of HIV encephalopathy, as well as a primary brain lymphoma. The patient died

Color Plates

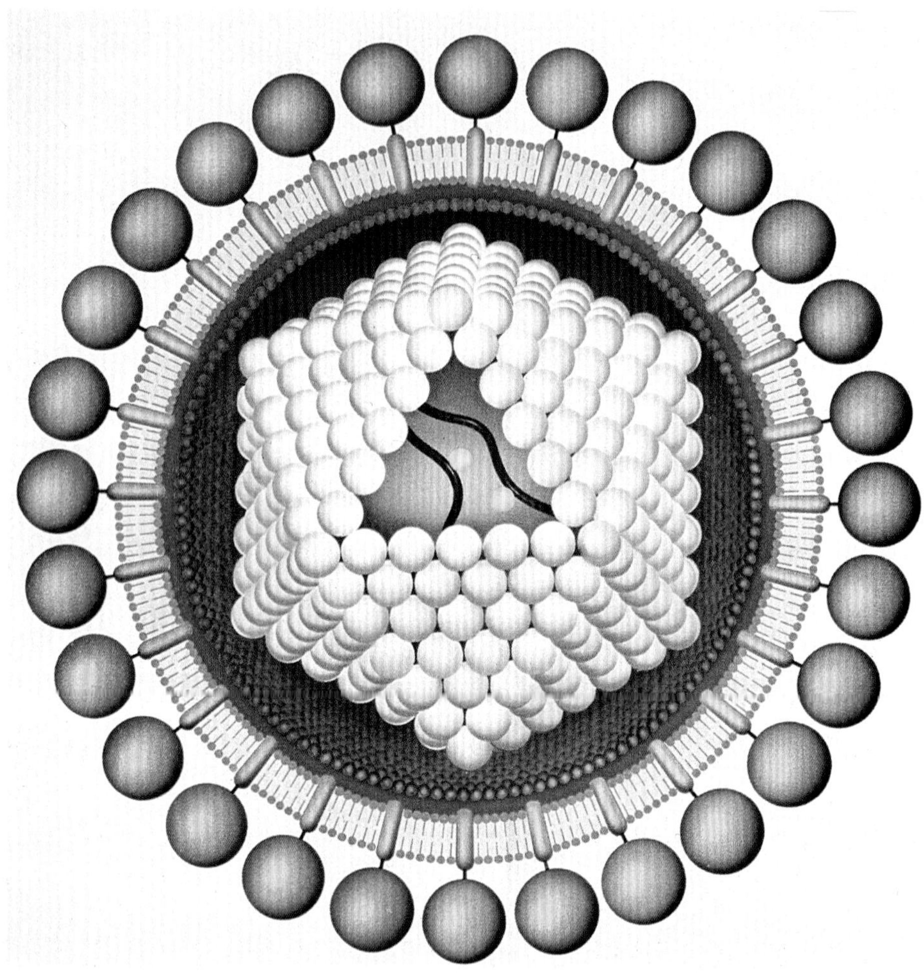

Plate 1-1. Schematic drawing of a retrovirus. The virus is about 1,000 angstrom units in diameter and consists of an inner nucleocapsid or core (extending to and including the brown elements) surrounded by an envelope (green and gray elements). The nucleocapsid contains two strands of RNA (red), multiple copies of reverse transcriptase (yellow) attached to the RNA, and associated core proteins (white and brown). The envelope is formed from a double lipid layer (gray) that is penetrated by surface glycoproteins (green). (From Gallo,[54] with permission.)

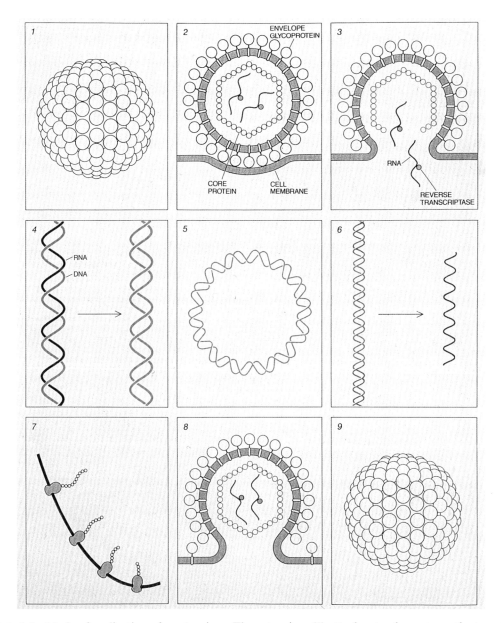

Plate 1-2. Mode of replication of a retrovirus. The retrovirus (1) attaches to elements on the target cell surface, (2) and the viral envelope fuses with the cell membrane (3). The viral RNA and its associated reverse transcriptase is released into the cell and a DNA copy (provirus) of the viral RNA is made (4) using the host cell's nucleotides. The viral RNA releases the single strand of DNA that has been made from it and a complementary DNA strand forms. This material probably migrates to the nucleus and circularizes (5). The DNA of some retroviruses is integrated into the host's chromosomes (6) and subsequently transcribed to RNA. Some of the RNA formed from the proviral DNA is translated into proteins in the cell cytoplasm by ribosomes (7). Viral RNA that is not translated associates with reverse transcriptase and nucleocapsid proteins made by the cellular ribosomes (8) and incorporates the host cell membrane as its envelope. Budding from the cell membrane, which is now permeated with viral glycoprotein components, allows formation of free viral particles (9). (From Gallo,[90] with permission.)

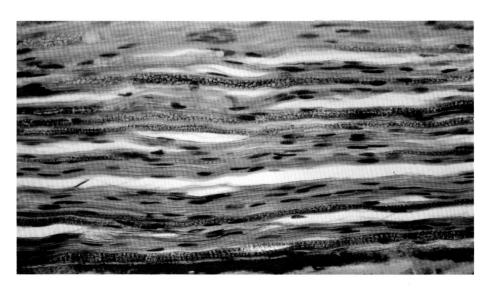

Plate 3-1. Longitudinal section of nerve in AIDS neuropathy. Myelin sheaths are stained red with this stain. Areas of fibrosis are green. There is considerable loss of myelin and, although this is not stained specifically for axons, presumably axons as well. (Trichrome stain, original magnification × 160.)

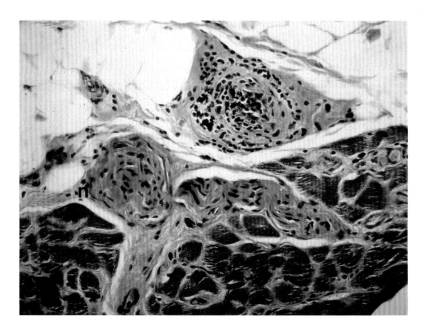

Plate 3-2. Vasculitis and neuropathy in muscle biopsy from a patient with AIDS. Muscle fibers (red), cut in cross section, are evident in the lower half of the section and a demyelinated fibrotic nerve (n) is evident at the edge of the muscle tissue. In the fat above the muscle there is a blood vessel with a mural mononuclear inflammatory infiltrate. (Gomorri trichrome stain, original magnification × 160.)

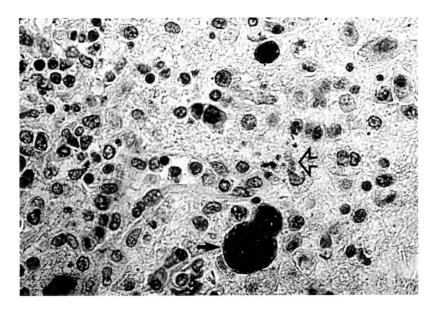

Plate 4-1. Immunohistochemical stain of toxoplasma organisms, both in pseudocysts (solid arrow-head) and free in the parenchyma (open arrowhead) of the pons. (Peroxidase-antiperoxidase stain, original magnification × 400.)

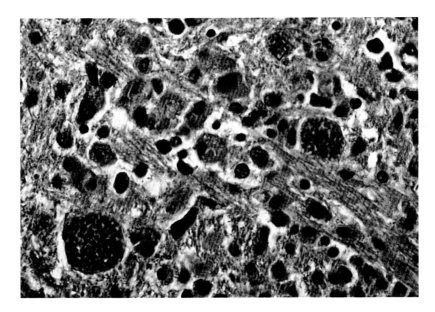

Plate 4-2. Toxoplasmosis in the brain stem. This microscopic section of the basis pontis includes three large toxoplasma pseudocysts (marked by diamonds) with associated inflammatory cells, which include histiocytes, plasma cells, and lymphocytes. (Hematoxylin and eosin stain, original magnification × 400.)

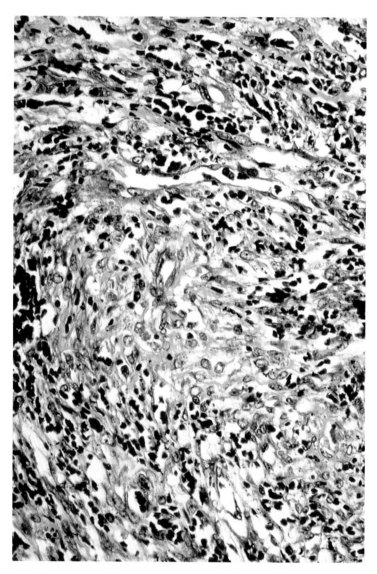

Plate 5-1. Kaposi's sarcoma. Metastatic tumor to the lung (original magnification × 250.)

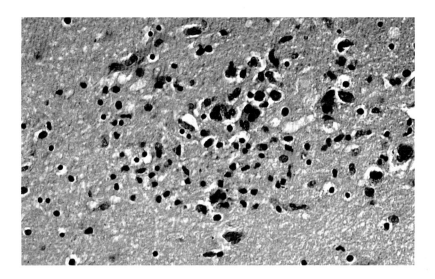

Plate 6-1. Microglial nodule in white matter in child with AIDS. There are two multinucleated giant cells in the center of the microglial nodule. (Hematoxylin and eosin stain, original magnification × 250.)

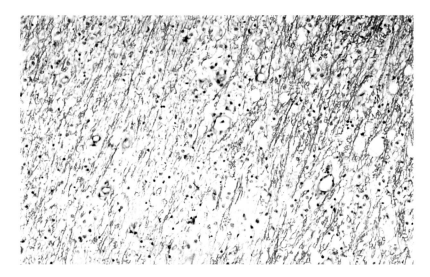

Plate 6-2. White matter in AIDS encephalopathy. Myelin is stained blue and appears normal at the upper right margin of the section. There is rarefaction and loss of myelin in most of the section examined. Blood vessels are stained pink. (Luxol fast blue/PAS stain, original magnification × 160.)

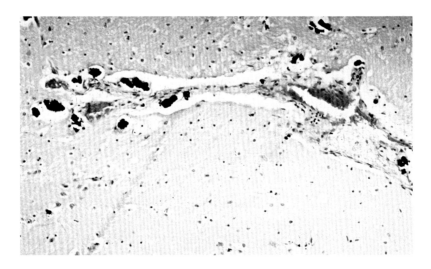

Plate 6-3. Perivascular calcifications in child with AIDS encephalopathy (original magnification × 160.)

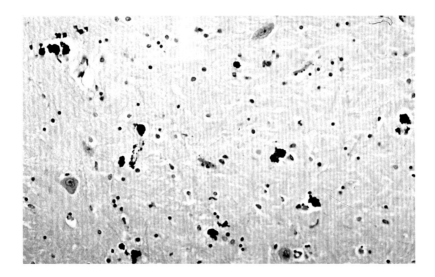

Plate 6-4. Calcifications in basal ganglia of child with AIDS (original magnification × 250.)

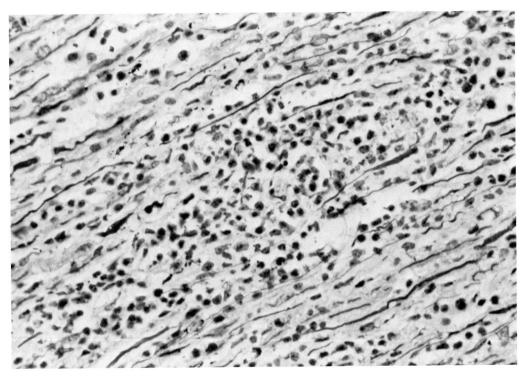

Fig. 5-1. Bodian stain of third cranial nerve infiltrated by lymphoma cells. The dark linear structures running diagonally are axons that are separated by the cellular infiltrate (original magnification × 160).

of vascular complications. As is often true in patients with AIDS, the diagnosis was suspected, but not demonstrable, until the autopsy. The patient's rapid deterioration frustrated efforts to identify and treat the intracranial problems.

Diagnosis

Computed tomography or MRI will reveal solitary or multiple lesions in the majority of affected individuals.[9,12,14] These lesions appear as low-density regions on CT.[8,15,16] Enchancement after contrast injection is usually present but is not usually prominent.[9,15] The entire lesion enhances slightly, except for areas of edema surrounding the tumor mass.[8] Masses of lymphoma tissue are usually situated in deep, periventricular locations.[17] Although the pattern of enhancement is usually distinct from that seen with toxoplasma granulomas, lymphomas cannot be reliably differentiated from toxoplasmosis on the basis of computed tomography.[8,17] Magnetic resonance imaging is no more likely to reveal or identify these brain lesions than computed tomography.

More invasive techniques may be helpful in establishing the diagnosis. Lumbar puncture is especially informative and is not associated with an increased incidence of herniation.[9] The cerebrospinal fluid is abnormal in more than 80 percent of affected individuals, the principal abnormalities being moderate elevations of the protein content and a mild pleocytosis.[9,12] Cells present in the spinal fluid are predominantly mononuclear and rarely exceed 40 cells per μL. The median cerebrospinal fluid protein content is 73 mg/dL.[9] The cerebrospinal fluid glucose is usually normal or slightly depressed.[9] Cytologic studies of the cerebrospinal fluid will rarely reveal clearly malignant cells, but the yield may be improved substantially by using large volumes of fluid collected with repeated spinal taps and stained with immunoperoxidase stains.[9,12] In most cases, brain biopsy is necessary for a definitive diagnosis.[4,9]

Histopathology

The lymphomas occurring in these immunosuppressed patients routinely form discrete tumor masses, rather than presenting as multiple small collections of tumor cells or as meningeal lymphomatosis. They usually arise from B lymphocytes and exhibit varied cellular morphology, including large cell immunoblastic and small noncleaved cell types[8,9] (Fig. 5-2). These are non-Hodgkin's lymphomas and have an unusually high incidence of high-grade histologic abnormalities.[9] The tumors consist of mixed cellular types, with transformed lymphoid cells intermixed with reactive small lymphocytes and mononuclear phagocytes.[9]

At autopsy, the lymphomas are often multifocal with indistinct borders and granular surfaces.[9] Tumors cluster along vascular channels. The spinal cord is usually spared, but leptomeningeal involvement is not unusual. Supratentorial tumors are more common than infratentorial tumors.[9] Primary brain lymphomas have been rare in infancy and childhood, but they do occur.

CASE HISTORY TWO

The male infant of an intravenous drug abusing mother was admitted at 1 month of age with pneumonia and evidence of cyto-

megalovirus in his urine. His mother was positive for HIV-1 antibodies, and he was found to have antibodies as well. Over the course of 4 months he recovered from the pneumonia and was discharged, but the pneumonia recurred and he was readmitted at 7 months of age. The pneumonia was treated with trimethoprim and sulfamethoxazole (Bactrim) on which he appeared to improve, but within a few weeks he developed low-grade fevers. At 8 months of age he had a generalized seizure, followed by a persistent left hemiparesis.

On evaluation of the hemiparesis, he was found to have bilateral optic atrophy, papilledema, and nystagmus. Hyperreflexia was evident bilaterally and ankle clonus occurred on the left. Cerebrospinal fluid protein was elevated to 270 mg/dL, but the sugar was normal. Cerebrospinal fluid cultures were consistently negative. Computed tomography of the brain revealed masses in the temporal and thalamic regions.

Chest roentgenograms revealed an interstitial infiltrate. Hepatosplenomegaly and inguinal lymphadenopathy were evident. His respiratory function deteriorated over the course of the next few weeks. He died at 10 months of age.

Examination of the brain at postmortem revealed a diffuse, small and large cell lymphoma, involving several regions of the brain. This was a primary brain lymphoma extending into both cerebral hemispheres and to a lesser extent the cerebellum. In the parenchyma of the brain, the cells were distributed in sheets with numerous focal accumulations. Both basal ganglia and the right thalamus contained tumor cells. Thalamic necrosis occurred along with the tumor infiltration (Fig. 5-3). Immunoperoxidase stains for B lymphocyte markers were uniformly negative. Associated with this lymphoma was cytomegalovirus infection of the ependyma, subependyma, and oculomotor nerves. Focal meningeal calcifications were evident along the spinal cord.

The immediate cause of death was bron-

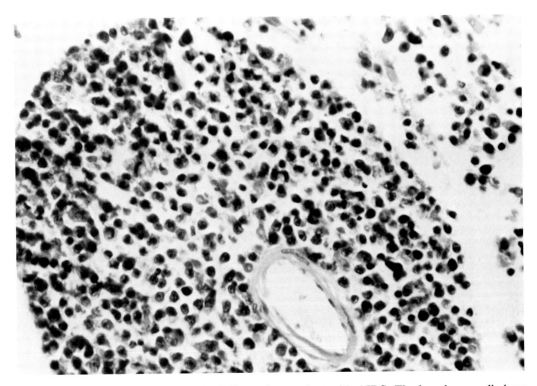

Fig. 5-2. Lymphomatous perivascular infiltrate in a patient with AIDS. The lymphoma cells have plasmacytoid features, such as slightly eccentric nuclei, and therefore probably originated from B lymphocytes. (Hematoxylin and eosin stain, original magnification ×250.)

chopneumonia with microabscess formation and pleuritis. This was the product of a chronic cytomegalovirus pneumonia. No bacteria or fungi were grown from the nervous system.

This infant had extensive central nervous system damage from a primary brain lymphoma and perinatal cytomegalovirus infection. The tumor was highly invasive and destructive, features that may be typical for primary lymphomas occurring this early in development or may be specific for this one individual. Too few primary brain lymphomas have been discovered in infants with AIDS to draw any conclusions except that primary brain lymphomas do occur in these patients as early as the first year of life. Primary brain lymphomas in adults are presumed to arise from B lymphocytes, but with a lesion arising perinatally or prena-

tally, cell markers may not conform to the adult pattern.

Pathophysiology

The lymphomas occurring in AIDS patients are usually immunoblastic sarcomas or plasmacytoid lymphocytic lymphomas.[8,18] These are both large cell tumors of B lymphocyte origin. They are lymphoproliferative malignancies that occur in other immune disorders and are not specific for HIV infection.[1,8]

Why lymphomas develop in the brain is unknown, but some blame neurotropic herpesviruses that gain access to the central nervous system in the immunosuppressed individual, and others suggest that there is special vulnerability to malignant transfor-

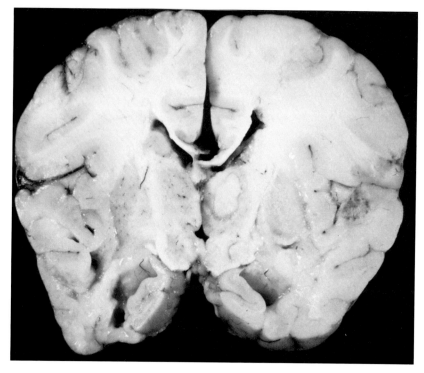

Fig. 5-3. Thalamic lesion in a 10-month-old boy representing primary brain lymphoma.

mation of brain lymphoid cells in these patients.[4,5] Gaining in credibility with extensive studies of genetic material in these tumors is that Epstein-Barr virus induces a B-cell lymphoproliferative disorder in AIDS patients.[19,20]

Patients with the Wiskott-Aldrich syndrome who develop CNS lymphomas account for about 25 percent of the population of patients who develop these tumors.[5] About 70 percent of the patients with primary CNS lymphomas have had vigorous immunosuppressive therapy with drugs, such as azathioprine and cyclophosphamide, to help them retain transplanted organs.[4,5,21] These immunosuppressive drugs do not cross the blood-brain barrier, so it is not obvious how they contribute to the development of primary brain tumors.

One mechanism postulated is that immunosuppressive drugs suppress peripheral B lymphocyte populations and thereby induce the production of excessive amounts of B cell colony stimulating hormone.[5,19] This excess colony stimulating hormone could cross the blood-brain barrier and induce inappropriate lymphocyte proliferation in the central nervous system.[5]

The lymphomas developing in the central nervous system in AIDS patients do appear to be B-cell lymphomas, but contrary to the model suggested for lymphomas arising with immunosuppression, patients with AIDS do not have depleted B-cell populations outside the central nervous system. The primary brain lymphomas arising with AIDS have features traditionally designated as immunoblastic or lymphoblastic, features that suggest that they may have undergone a malignant transformation in response to an infecting virus.[22]

That a virus is truly responsible has not been demonstrated, but some investigators believe that the Epstein-Barr virus will prove to induce the malignant transformation.[5,23] The Epstein-Barr virus clearly can infect and immortalize B lymphocytes in culture.[23] If this occurred in the central nervous system of the patient with AIDS, the immortal B lymphocytes could develop autonomous clones, that is, individual cell types that would reproduce outside the restraints usually limiting B lymphocyte proliferation.[8,24] Outside the central nervous system, the immune system, even in the severely impaired AIDS patient, is probably adequately competent to destroy these aberrant cells as soon as they appear.[8] In the brain, lymphomas develop because the central nervous system has a distinct system of immune surveillance, a system that is apparently more permissive when it comes to abnormal B lymphocytes.[8] The immortal lymphocyte survives in this sequestered environment, and the clone that results produces tumors.

Treatment

Primary brain lymphomas usually become apparent at a very advanced stage and exhibit a poor response to therapy.[9] Survival from the time of diagnosis is often limited to weeks.[8] Surgical resection serves little purpose, since the tumors are usually multifocal at a microscopic level, if not at a gross level.

Whole brain irradiation may suppress or eliminate a primary brain lymphoma, but the course of treatment requires weeks, rather than days, a feature of the treatment that limits its usefulness in rapidly deteriorating patients.[25] Most radiation protocols use 5,000 rads to the brain or the entire craniospinal axis to suppress the tumor.[8,25]

Even if the tumor does respond favorably to radiation, the patients are at very high risk of opportunistic infections.[26]

Concurrent treatment with systemic chemotherapy is often attempted.[8] Cyclophosphamide, melphalan, vincristine, and prednisone have been used in combination in some patients.[8] Other antineoplastic regimens include bleomycin and doxorubicin. That any regimen has advantages over another remains to be demonstrated.

The prognosis is poor even with aggressive treatment. With radiosensitive lymphomas and appropriate radiation, the average survival from the time of diagnosis is only 2 months.[9] This is more the result of systemic problems at the time of diagnosis than from the central nervous system tumor itself.[9] Patients with brain lymphomas usually die from refractory pneumonia and sepsis. Those who survive for a full course of cranial irradiation do exhibit regression of the tumor.[9]

METASTATIC LYMPHOMAS

Patients with HIV infection occasionally develop systemic lymphomas that metastasize to the central nervous system.[12] Because the diagnosis of AIDS presumes there is no systemic basis for immunodeficiency such as a disseminated lymphoma, there are semantic objections to designating these patients as AIDS victims. Meningeal lymphomatosis may develop with these systemic lymphomas and occasionally epidural collections cause spinal cord compression.[12] The outlook with these lymphomas is considerably better than that with primary central nervous system lymphomas, survival extending to months, rather than weeks.[12]

KAPOSI'S SARCOMA

Early after the appearance of AIDS in the homosexual population, an unusually aggressive form of Kaposi's sarcoma was described in both homosexuals and intravenous drug abusers.[3,27–29] Before the AIDS epidemic, Kaposi's sarcoma was not generally found in patients under 50 years of age and was rarely lethal.[3,28,30] The median age of men with opportunistic infections and Kaposi's sarcoma was 35 in a survey conducted by the Centers for Disease Control before the significance of the connection to AIDS was fully appreciated.[3] Most of those affected before the AIDS epidemic were men of Eastern European descent or renal allograft recipients.[30] From the earliest reports of the sharp rise in the incidence of Kaposi's sarcoma, the connection to communities of homosexual men was apparent.[3,31] The previously rare metastatic Kaposi's sarcoma initially appeared to have a predilection for homosexual men who developed AIDS, but it is now evident that all high risk groups developing AIDS may develop this tumor.[3] The link to immunosuppression was assumed because of the concurrent appearance of opportunistic infections in many of the men affected. That Kaposi's sarcoma developed with unusual frequency in immunosuppressed patients was already apparent from the experience with organ recipients maintained on immunosuppressants.[3]

Signs and Symptoms

The sarcoma is manifest superficially as a violaceous nodule or patch.[31,32] These lesions may be fairly inconspicuous and may remain undetected because of their location in mucous membranes.[3] In biopsied lymph nodes, patients with Kaposi's sarcoma may exhibit a dense proliferation of spindle-shaped cells that extend irregularly in many directions[27] (Fig. 5-4, Plate 5-1). There are usually foci of grouped capillaries of various sizes.

Kaposi's sarcoma apparently can metastasize to the brain in patients with or without AIDS.[12,33,34] The brain masses are likely to be hemorrhagic. Metastatic tumors have also been described involving the brachial plexus and resulting in a plexopathy.[12]

Etiology

Before the connection between AIDS and Kaposi's sarcoma was appreciated, some investigators postulated that a cytomegalovirus infection was triggering or contributing to the development of the tumor.[30] CMV antigens or genomes can often be isolated from Kaposi's sarcoma tissue, but conclusive evidence that CMV actually produced the tumor has always been lacking.[30]

This tumor is apparently not a direct effect of sarcomatous tissue infection with the human immunodeficiency virus. Rather, it appears to develop in response to growth factors released by infected lymphocytes. The sarcoma may in fact not be a conventional malignancy, but this will be more apparent when strategies to interfere with the growth factors have been developed.

Treatment

The appearance of Kaposi's sarcoma is not a grave sign. This tumor is sensitive to radiation therapy, and individuals with this problem alone are likely to do well.[12,34] Patients with AIDS who have manifested Kaposi's sarcoma alone as their principal problem are only one-fourth as likely to have succumbed to their disease as individuals who have developed pneumocystis pneumonia.[3]

OTHER TUMORS

Despite continued surveillance for the appearance of other tumors in AIDS, no other

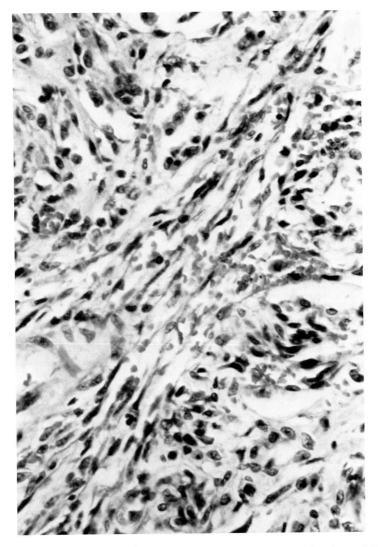

Fig. 5-4. Kaposi's sarcoma. Primary nodule (original magnification ×250).

malignancies have developed with the extraordinary frequency of lymphoma and Kaposi's sarcoma. As survival increases, it is probable that other tumors will develop. The reticuloendothelial system is apparently at special risk, so lymphomatous lesions inside and outside the nervous system will probably be seen.

REFERENCES

1. CDC: Revision of the CDC surveillance case definition for acquired immunodeficiency syndrome. MMWR 36:3s, 1987
2. Guarda LA, Luna MA, Smith JL, et al: AIDS: postmortem findings. Am J Clin Pathol 81:549, 1984

3. Centers for Disease Control Task Force on Kaposi's Sarcoma and Opportunistic Infections: Epidemiologic aspects of the current outbreak of Kaposi's sarcoma and opportunistic infections. N Engl J Med 306:248, 1982

4. Snider WD, Simpson DM, Aronyk KE, Nielsen SL: Primary lymphoma of the nervous system associated with acquired immune-deficiency syndrome. N Engl J Med 308:45, 1983

5. Kay HEM: Immunosuppression and the risk of brain lymphoma. N Engl J Med 308:1099, 1983

6. Kotasek D, Albertyn LE, Sage RE: A five-year experience with central nervous system lymphoma. Med J Aust 144:299, 1986

7. Levitt LJ: CNS involvement in the non-Hodgkin's lymphomas. Cancer 95:545, 1980

8. Gill PS, Levine AM, Meyer PR, et al: Primary central nervous system lymphoma in homosexual men. Am J Med 78:742, 1985

9. So YT, Beckstead HJ, Davis RL: Primary central nervous system lymphoma in acquired immune deficiency syndrome: a clinical and pathological study. Ann Neurol 20:566, 1986

10. Freeman CR, Shustik C, Brisson M-L, et al: Primary malignant lymphoma of the CNS. Cancer 58:1106, 1986

11. Levine AM, Gill PS, Meyer PR, et al: Retrovirus and malignant lymphoma in homosexual men. JAMA 254:1921, 1985

12. Levy RM, Bredesen DE, Rosenblum ML: Neurologic manifestations of the acquired immunodeficiency syndrome (AIDS): experience at the University of California at San Francisco and review of the literature. J Neurosurg 62:475, 1985

13. Case 31-1987: A 50-year-old woman with a central nervous system disorder and renal failure two months after renal transplantation. N Engl J Med 317:295, 1987

14. Anders KH, Guerra WF, Tomiyasu U, et al: The neuropathology of AIDS. UCLA experience and review. Am J Pathol 124:537, 1986

15. Mendenhall NP, Thar TL, Agee OF, et al: Primary lymphoma of the central nervous system. Computerized tomography scan characteristics and treatment results for 12 cases. Cancer 52:1993, 1983

16. Spillane JA, Kendall BE, Moseley IF: Cerebral lymphoma: clinical radiological correlation. J Neurol Neurosurg Psychiatry 45:199, 1982

17. Elkin CM, Leon E, Grenell SL, Leeds NE: Intracranial lesions in acquired immunodeficiency syndrome. JAMA 253:393, 1985

18. Levine AM, Meyer PR, Bagandy MK, et al: Development of B-cell lymphoma in homosexual men: Clinical and immunologic findings. Ann Intern Med 100:7, 1984

19. Shearer WT, Ritz J, Finegold MJ, et al: E-B virus associated B cell proliferation of diverse clonal origins after bone marrow transplantation in a 12-year-old patient with severe combined immunodeficiency. N Engl J Med 312:1151, 1985

20. Case 9-1986: A 40-month-old girl with the acquired immunodeficiency syndrome and spinal-cord compression. N Engl J Med 314:629, 1986

21. Frizzera G, Rosai J, Dehner LP, et al: Lymphoreticular disorders in primary immunodeficiency; new findings based on an up to date histologic classification of 35 cases. Cancer 46:692, 1980

22. Reichert CM, O'Leary TJ, Levens DL, et al: Autopsy pathology in the acquired immune deficiency syndrome. Am J Pathol 112:357, 1983

23. Klein G: Lymphoma development in mice and humans: diversity of initiation is followed by convergent cytogenetic evolution. Proc Natl Acad Sci USA 76:2442, 1979

24. Cleary ML, Warnke R, Sklar J: Monoclonality of lymphoproliferative lesions in cardiac-transplant recipients; clonal analysis based on immunoglobulin-gene rearrangements. N Engl J Med 310:477, 1984

25. Berry MP, Simpson WJ: Radiation therapy in the management of primary malignant lymphoma of the brain. Int J Radiat Oncol Biol Phys 7:55–59, 1981

26. Snow RB, Lavyne MH: Intracranial space-occupying lesions in acquired immunodeficiency syndrome patients. Neurosurgery (Baltimore) 16:148, 1985

27. Gold KD, Thomas L, Garrett TJ: Aggressive Kaposi's sarcoma in a heterosexual drug addict. N Engl J Med 307:498, 1982

28. Hymes KB, Cheung T, Greene JB, et al: Kaposi's sarcoma in homosexual men—a report of eight cases. Lancet 2:598, 1981

29. Koziner B, Denny T, Myskowski PL, et al: Opportunistic infections and Kaposi's sarcoma in homosexual men. N Engl J Med 306:933, 1982

30. Drew WL, Conant MA, Miner RC, et al: Cytomegalovirus and Kaposi's sarcoma in young homosexual men. lancet 2:125, 1982

31. Barton NW, Safai B, Nielson SL, Posner JB: Neurological complications of Kaposi's sarcoma: an analysis of 5 cases and a review of the literature. Neurooncology 1:333, 1983

32. Vilaseca J, Arnau JM, Bacardi R, et al: Kaposi's sarcoma and *Toxoplasma gondii* brain abscess in a Spanish homosexual. Lancet 1:572, 1982

33. Rwomushana RJW, Bailey JC, Kyalwazi SK: Kaposi's sarcoma of the brain. Cancer 36:1127, 1975

34. Levy RM, Pons VG, Rosenblum ML: Intracerebral mass lesions in the acquired immunodeficiency syndrome (AIDS). J Neurosurg 61:9, 1984

6

Neurologic Disease in Infants and Children

Although the manifestations of the acquired immune deficiency syndrome (AIDS) in children and infants share many features with the syndrome observed in adults, several features not seen in adults are typical or common in infants and children. What constitutes AIDS in infants and children has been repeatedly revised as features of the syndrome that are not seen in adults have become more evident.[1-3] The child with HIV infection has AIDS if multiple or recurrent serious bacterial infections occur, even if the bacteria involved are not opportunistic.[1] Also, the coexistence of HIV infection and lymphoid interstitial hyperplasia, an excessive cellular infiltrate into the tissues of both lungs, is diagnostic of AIDS in the child, yet not observed in adults.[1] Kaposi's sarcoma and other phenomena commonly seen in adults with AIDS have not yet been described in infants and children with AIDS.

Problems that by definition can only occur in childhood, such as failure to thrive and developmental regressions, are also routinely seen in children with AIDS. This is not surprising since growth and development are often affected by severe infections, regardless of the cause. What is surprising is that progressive encephalopathy occurs in children with no signs of opportunistic infections and few or no signs of

immune deficiency.[4] Cognitive development is especially vulnerable because central nervous system disease can appear in these children with either opportunistic infections or HIV damage to the brain. Infants and children with HIV infection often exhibit a progressive or static encephalopathy.[5] As in adults it is difficult to ascertain whether neurologic damage is directly from the human immunodeficiency virus or from concurrent infections given access to the nervous system by the immunodeficiency syndrome.[2,6]

Whether the affected child has direct involvement of the brain with HIV, damage to the central nervous system from opportunistic infections, or both, there is likely to be a failure to thrive, developmental regression, or death from overwhelming infections during the first few months or years after symptoms appear.[7] Normal growth and development will be disturbed with either a progressive encephalopathy or a static encephalopathy. Children with AIDS die months or years after symptoms of the HIV infection first appear.

ACQUISITION OF AIDS

The most common route for acquisition of the virus by the infant is from an infected mother across the placenta.[7-9] Most of the

111

women bearing children who develop AIDS have AIDS or signs of HIV infection, but the woman transmitting the disease to the fetus need not be symptomatic during the pregnancy.[7,10] Women bearing HIV-infected children have been predominantly intravenous drug abusers, the sexual partners of intravenous drug abusers or bisexual men, or Haitians.[11–13] Haitian women presumably acquire the disease through heterosexual activity. There is no indication that one high risk group is more likely to transmit the disease to its fetuses than any other. The only precondition for transmitting AIDS to the fetus is that the mother harbors human immunodeficiency virus. There is no evidence that HIV infection in the father has any bearing on the risk of infection faced by the fetus, except to the extent that the risk of infection in the mother is increased.

Even after testing for antibodies to the AIDS virus was widely available, infants and children still occasionally acquired the virus through blood transfusions.[10,14,15] Infants who do not receive transfusions rarely acquire the infection after birth, but isolated cases have been reported. Transmission of HIV through breast milk has been postulated to explain some cases.[16,17] Although sexual transmission of HIV to the infant or child is rare, it may occur and is usually an indication of child abuse.

That a child has acquired HIV in utero is difficult to document because of the maternal response to HIV infection.[18] Mothers infected with the retrovirus produce IgG antibodies that are transferred to the fetus across the placenta.[1,18] Passively acquired maternal antibodies to HIV may persist in the infant's blood for many months.[1] Consequently, blood taken from the umbilical cord of the newborn will test positive for antibodies to HIV by ELISA or Western Blot in virtually all cases in which the mother tests positive.[18] This does not indicate that the retrovirus has actually infected the infant; that can only be estab-

lished by isolating the virus or viral antigens from the child's tissues or demonstrating that the newborn has produced its own IgM antibodies to HIV, both of which are technically difficult.[18] In many cases, prenatal or perinatal acquisition of HIV can only be presumed from the subsequent development of AIDS in the infant. Unfortunately, the rate of transmission of HIV from infected mothers to their fetuses prenatally or perinatally is in excess of 60 percent and may be close to 100 percent.[19,20]

The majority of hemophiliacs who have developed AIDS are children.[14,21] As discussed in Chapter 2, hemophiliacs have acquired HIV through the use of pooled blood products. Even with rigorous testing for antibodies to HIV antigens in the pooled blood products that these children require, some virus occasionally gets transmitted to the child unless heat treatment or other procedures are followed.[10,14] The transmission of HIV is less likely as techniques for detecting antibodies to HIV become more rigorous, but most of the children with hemophilia who require transfusions of blood or blood products have acquired HIV already.

Close contact with children infected with HIV has yet to produce cases of AIDS in playmates, siblings, or parents.[22] This is reassuring to those who wish to avoid isolating these infected children and is consistent with current ideas about how the virus is transmitted. However, many physicians believe that the experience with HIV has been too brief to assume that the issue is settled. If the virus can produce infection with protracted, but not sexual, contact with infected individuals, cases of AIDS should start appearing in the families of infected children within the next few years.

Theories on how AIDS is acquired in infants and children presume that HIV can have an exceedingly long incubation period.[4] The offspring of women with HIV infection may develop signs and symptoms of AIDS months to years after birth.[3,4] For those children who were not nursed or sexually abused, the virus is presumed to have been transmitted transplacentally. This presumes that the virus may do little for 5 years and then cause a lethal illness. The alternative is to assume that the child acquires the virus months or years after birth through unrecognized mechanisms.

SOURCES OF DIAGNOSTIC CONFUSION

In infants and children, ascertaining that AIDS is responsible for developmental delays, developmental regression, congenital brain damage, or even immunodeficiency may be difficult. Prenatally acquired infections other than HIV encephalopathy may produce extensive neurologic damage in the developing fetus, and many of these intrauterine infections are caused by the same agents that appear in infants with AIDS. Further confusing the diagnosis of AIDS is the early onset of symptoms in many congenital immunodeficiency states that are unrelated to HIV infection. Early recognition of what is not AIDS is valuable in planning treatment and estimating prognosis.

Non-AIDS Immunodeficiency

Immunodeficiency develops in infants and children with hereditary disorders and acquired disease (Table 6-1). The more complex syndromes, such as DiGeorge, Wiskott-Aldrich, and ataxia telangiectasia are the easiest to distinguish because problems other than immunodeficiency belie the source of the problem. In ataxia telangiectasia, cerebellar signs usually precede symptoms of immune dysfunction by years, and the immunoglobulin levels are low, rather than inappropriately high, as is often true with AIDS.[23] Idiopathic gammopathies and neutropenias also have patterns of white blood cell disturbances that are distinct from AIDS. In some of these congenital immunodeficiencies, the normal development of T lymphocytes or other cellular elements of the immune system is blocked, and so mature active cells are not apparent.[10] In children with AIDS, these cells are present, but the deficiency in CD4 (helper-inducer) T lymphocytes is evident.[10] Even if the child has been exposed to immunosuppressive drugs and exhibits a secondary immunodeficiency, the characteristic selective depletion of helper-inducer T lymphocytes invariably seen in AIDS will not be evident.[24]

CYTOMEGALIC INCLUSION DISEASE

Cytomegalic inclusion disease is caused by cytomegalovirus and may have many features in common with AIDS when it occurs prenatally or perinatally[25] (Table 6-2). Complicating the differentiation of AIDS from cytomegalic disease is their frequent coexistence: Infants with congenital AIDS are at high risk of developing CMV encephalitis. Infants with severe CMV infec-

Table 6-1. Non-AIDS Causes of Immunodeficiency in Infants and Children

Primary	Secondary
DiGeorge syndrome	Immunosuppressive
Wiskott-Aldrich	therapy
syndrome	Lymphoreticular
Ataxia-telangiectasia	malignancy
Graft-versus-host disease	Malnutrition
Idiopathic gammopathies	
Idiopathic neutropenia	

Table 6-2. Neurologic Manifestations of Prenatal CMV Infection

Clinical	Pathologic
Seizures	Microcephaly
Mental retardation	Optic atrophy
Hemiparesis or	Chorioretinitis
quadriparesis	Polymicrogyria
Sensorineural deafness	Cerebellar atrophy
Visual impairment	Periventricular
	calcifications
	Microglial nodules

tion exhibit hepatitis, splenomegaly, pneumonia, thrombocytopenia, chorioretinitis, and extensive neurologic damage as a consequence of the CMV infection.[25] Neonates with extensive brain damage from CMV may have seizures, spasticity, blindness, and developmental delays.[25] Objective neurologic changes associated with congenital CMV infection include microcephaly, polymicrogyria, cerebellar hypoplasia, and optic atrophy, as well as chorioretinitis.

Microglial nodules occur in reaction to either CMV or HIV infection of the brain, but as noted in Chapter 4, the nodules with CMV are more strictly periventricular than those occurring with HIV. Calcifications may occur in the basal ganglia of infants with prenatal infection, a pathologic feature shared with congenital HIV encephalopathy.[25] Helpful in distinguishing between AIDS and CMV is evidence of cytomegalic infection outside the nervous system, with inclusion bodies in the nuclei and cytoplasm of affected cells.[25]

SIGNS AND SYMPTOMS OF AIDS

The more typical features of AIDS, such as lymphadenopathy, diarrhea, candidiasis, hepatosplenomegaly, and *Pneumocystis carinii* pneumonia, develop with the same regularity in infants and children as in adults[10,15,26] (Table 6-3). Parotitis and recurrent bacterial infections with organisms

Table 6-3. Systemic Disease in Children with AIDS

Disorder	Percent Affected
Chronic interstitial pneumonitis	100
Hepatosplenomegaly	97
Failure to thrive	94
Diffuse adenopathy	56
Protracted or recurrent diarrhea	39
Thrombocytopenia	31
Low birth weight (less than 2,500 gm)	28
Eczemoid rash	19
Recurrent otitis media	19

Based on data from Shannon et al.[24]

that are not, strictly speaking, opportunistic are seen much more often in children and infants than in adults.[7] Virtually all children and infants with AIDS will exhibit hepatosplenomegaly, interstitial pneumonitis, and poor growth.[24] Most will have frequent bouts of diarrhea, otitis media, and rashes.[24] *Pneumocystis carinii* pneumonia occurs in more than one-third of the children who develop AIDS.[24]

Immunologic studies early in the course of disease in infected infants reveal a polyclonal hypergammaglobulinemia, much like that seen in adults.[15,24] This apparently results from unregulated B lymphocyte clones.[27,28] Immunodeficiency is also manifest by a decrease in the absolute number of helper-inducer (CD4) T lymphocytes (less than 1000/μL of peripheral blood) and a helper/suppressor ratio of less than 1.0.[4] The thymus in the infant with AIDS will be hypoplastic and the T lymphocyte abnormalities characteristic of affected adults will be apparent.[15] Boys and girls are equally likely to be affected.[4]

Reduction of the helper/suppressor ratio to less than 1.0 is a less reliable indicator of AIDS in children than in adults because opportunistic Epstein-Barr virus or cytomegalovirus infections can cause a similar shift in the ratio.[24] Indeed, this T4/T8 (CD4/CD8) ratio is also less useful in children than in adults because it not only may be depressed by non-AIDS viral infections, but is frequently greater than 1.0 in children who unequivocally have AIDS.[24]

In children with HIV-1 antibodies, a lymphoid interstitial pneumonitis has become virtually diagnostic of AIDS[29] (Table 6-4). This infiltrating lesion in the lungs produces a reticulonodular pattern on the chest x-ray; the children exhibit cough and dyspnea.[29] Infants may exhibit persistent lymphadenopathy or mild immune dysfunction without developing AIDS until months or possibly years after acquiring the virus. Autoimmune disease with associated thrombocytopenia and a non-iron defi-

Table 6-4. Characteristics of AIDS in Infancy and Childhood

Transmission	In utero
	Through breast milk
	Transfusions
	Sexual abuse
Signs and symptoms	Lymphoid interstitial hyperplasia
	Opportunistic infections
	Progressive encephalopathy or static encephalopathy
Age at onset	2 months to 5 years (if acquired in utero)
Mortality	Probably 100 percent in 8 years

ciency anemia can occur in infants with HIV infection who do not exhibit AIDS.[15,29] The prognosis for these children is unknown.

Kaposi's sarcoma is notably uncommon in children with AIDS.[29] Even the perennial *Toxoplasma gondii* threat to the central nervous system that exacts so large a toll in adult populations is of relatively minor importance in pediatric populations, probably because few of the children with AIDS have adequate environmental exposure to acquire the protozoan. Epstein-Barr virus infections, however, as evidenced by antibody production to this virus, are exceedingly common in infants.[7] Serious bacterial infections and recurrent bacteremia with streptococci and staphylococci are much more common in children with AIDS than in adults with AIDS.[24] Pneumococcal sepsis may be fatal in these children.[29] The majority will exhibit candidal infections early in the course of their disease.[24]

Developmental Delays

At least half of the children who have HIV infection develop a progressive encephalopathy[4] (Table 6-5). These children need not have signs of immunosuppression; however, all children with HIV infection and immunosuppression exhibit abnormalities in development. Delays in achieving motor milestones are the most obvious deficiencies.[4] Older children exhibit perceptual problems, and if language disturbances occur, they appear to be predominantly expressive, rather than receptive.[6] The neurologic deterioration may be stepwise in progression, so the child may appear to stabilize for months at a time. Neurologic deterioration between quiescent periods usually lasts a few weeks at the most.[4] The intermittent stabilization exhibited by these children will complicate clinical trials of anti-HIV drugs, but it appears that all children with progressive encephalopathy die.[2,4]

With the static encephalopathy associated with exposure to HIV, the child may exhibit developmental delays or nonprogressive motor deficits.[5] Children with static encephalopathies do not have signs of active central nervous system infection with HIV, such as intrablood-brain barrier production of antibodies against the virus.[5] That the encephalopathy is permanently static in these children will become more evident over the next few years.

Developmental Regression

With progressive encephalopathy, the child is likely to exhibit developmental regression if development has proceeded past some early milestones at the time that the infection becomes symptomatic.[5] Brain growth will slow measurably with progressive encephalopathy.[5,7] Microcephaly may be apparent.[7] This arrest of gross brain growth is less likely with a static encephalopathy.

Children with HIV infection and a progressive encephalopathy usually exhibit loss of developmental milestones or intellectual ability, progressive limb weakness and spasticity, and hyperreflexia.[5] Babinski signs may reappear. Some children develop ataxia, extrapyramidal rigidity, and seizures.[5,7] Progressive encephalopathy in children with HIV infection is almost certainly from brain damage inflicted by the

Table 6-5. Findings with HIV Encephalopathy in Children

Clinical		Structural
Common	Occasional	
Loss of milestones	Extrapyramidal rigidity	Atrophy on MR or CT
Bilateral spasticity	Dysarthria	Reduced head circumference in infants
Ataxia	Dysphagia	Hydrocephalus ex vacuo
Hypertonia or hypotonia	Seizures	Basal ganglia calcifications
Paraparesis or quadriparesis		
Myoclonic jerks		

retrovirus itself.[4,5] For progressive encephalopathy to occur in AIDS, HIV must be expressed and probably must be replicating within the central nervous system of the affected child.[2,5]

Moro or tonic neck reflexes may persist in affected children past 4 months of age.[4] Symmetric ankle clonus and extensor plantar responses are evident early in the course of clinical deterioration in older children. Pseudobulbar palsy, dysphagia, and dysarthria develop as the affected child develops a spastic quadriparesis. Some children develop myoclonic jerks independent of periodic discharges on the EEG.[4]

Neurodiagnostic Studies

Structural changes in the brain are evident on routine clinical investigations. MRI or CT will reveal a secondary microcephaly in those children with early onset disease. Serial measurements of head circumference will also establish impaired brain growth if there is a progressive encephalopathy. Associated with the atrophy, is increased ventricular size and enlargement of sulcal markings, changes usually referred to as hydrocephalus ex vacuo.[4,5] Bilateral symmetric calcifications occur in many infants and children with HIV encephalopathy, a finding not at all characteristic of the HIV subacute encephalitis seen in the adult.[4] Periventricular white matter, as well as the basal ganglia, may have calcifications but this is less common.[4] No edema is associated with this calcification, but contrast en-

hancement in the basal ganglia may be evident on CT.[4]

Cerebrospinal fluid studies are often quite unrevealing in the child with HIV encephalopathy.[4] If the white cell count is at all increased, it is usually by less than 20 cells/μL, and all of these cells are likely to be lymphocytes. The protein content of the fluid is normal or slightly increased to less than 80 mg/dL. Other cerebrospinal fluid parameters, such as glucose content and cultures, are routinely normal.

Antibodies to HIV are produced within the central nervous system of infected children.[2,4,5] Some of these are neutralizing antibodies, a distinction of considerable importance, at least in children, since individuals without neutralizing antibodies have a much more rapid deterioration. Failure to detect such antibodies does not prove that HIV infection has not occurred.

PROGNOSIS

The average interval from onset of progressive neurologic signs to death is about 8 months for infants and children.[4,5,7] If the child with HIV antibody proof of exposure to the AIDS virus has a static encephalopathy or no neurologic problems, survival is unpredictable.[4] If antibodies to the AIDS virus are found at levels high enough in the cerebrospinal fluid to indicate that they were formed within the nervous system itself, then the prognosis for the untreated child is grim.[5] Progressive encephalopathy over the course of months or years will usually appear with brain involvement by the virus.

Whether AIDS is invariably lethal in children who become symptomatic is unknown. Three-year survival is less than 25 percent.[24] Five-year survival without anti-HIV therapy may be close to 0 percent. Experience with this disease in children is too brief to exclude the possibility of survival in some cases. There is at least one report from Africa of a child with AIDS who survived after evidence of disease in the first year of life.[30] At 7 years of age, the child was allegedly healthy and neurologically intact. The child's mother died of AIDS.[30]

The experience with AIDS in children in the United States and Europe has not been at all encouraging. Children with HIV infection develop AIDS months or years after acquiring the virus and die within months or years after developing AIDS.[5,7] The delay from date of acquisition of the virus until the appearance of progressive neurologic deficits may be as brief as 2 months or as long as 5 years.[4]

NEUROPATHOLOGIC FEATURES

Pathologic findings in the pediatric victim of HIV subacute encephalitis are similar to those seen in adults (Table 6-6). The brain is small for age but otherwise often appears grossly normal. The multinucleated giant or syncytial cell typical of HIV encephalopathy is usually evident, but even more ob-

Table 6-6. Neuropathologic Findings in Children with HIV Encephalopathy

Microscopic	Gross
Vascular calcification	Decreased brain weight
White matter pallor or astrocytosis	Small for age
Inflammatory cell infiltrates	
Multinucleated giant cells	
Vascular inflammation	

vious in the pediatric brain is perivascular calcification,[2,4] which is usually present in the basal ganglia.

Inflammatory cell infiltrates consist of microglial cells, lymphocytes, and plasma cells, as well as the multinucleated giant cell[4,7] (Fig. 6-1). These infiltrates are widespread but most commonly are found in deep structures of the basal ganglia and brain stem.[2,4] Inflammatory cell infiltrates and multinucleated giant cells have been reported as being more evident in the brains of children with HIV infection than in the brains of adults[2,3] (Plate 6-1). The vacuolar myelopathy so commonly seen in adults is rare, if not in fact nonexistent, in children.[31] Conversely, the perivascular calcifications evident in the brains of children are generally not seen in the brains of affected adults.

White matter changes include pallor and astrocytosis.[4] The demyelination described in adult lesions is not prominent in pediatric cases (Plate 6-2). Opportunistic infections, such as toxoplasmosis and cryptococcosis, which are routinely seen in adults with HIV infection of the brain, are also not evident.[2-4] The microglial nodules and Cowdry type A inclusions associated with cerebral cytomegalovirus infection are evident in some children's brains (Fig 6-2).

Case History One

A 2-year-old baby girl was admitted in 1987 for evaluation of fever and hematemesis. Three years earlier her father had traveled from Brazil to New York City where he allegedly acquired AIDS. He returned to Brazil before he was symptomatic and transmitted the disease to his wife. Shortly thereafter, he developed progressive dementia and Kaposi's sarcoma. His wife became pregnant after his return from New York and had an apparently healthy baby girl. The pregnancy and delivery were uncomplicated, but the child soon devel-

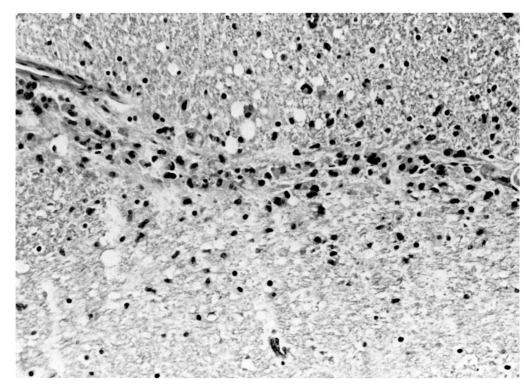

Fig. 6-1. AIDS encephalopathy in a child. This autopsy specimen from the pons of a 9-year-old boy with AIDS encephalopathy shows the characteristic perivascular microglial infiltrate and vacuolation of myelin. (Hematoxylin and eosin stain, original magnification ×160.)

oped hepatitis and toxoplasmosis and was found to be HIV positive. The mother was also HIV positive, but both continued in fairly good health until the child was about 1 year of age. The child's father died of complications of AIDS.

Both mother and child came to New York City from Brazil. The mother soon developed *Pneumocystis carinii* pneumonia, but the child continued to exhibit normal growth and development throughout the first year of life. At that point the child developed failure to thrive and regression of developmental milestones. Within a few months of her first birthday, she developed seizures.

On examination the child's head circumference was below the fifth percentile, as were her height and weight. She had a fever but no heart murmurs. On admission she

was already unconscious, with no response to visual or auditory stimuli. Her pupils were fixed and slightly dilated. She had purposeless writhing movements with occasional decerebrate posturing on the day of admission.

The patient was treated with ceftriaxone and nasogastric feedings. She defervesced initially, but 5 days after hospitalization, she developed recurrent hematemesis and fever. Two days later she had respiratory distress secondary to unexplained pneumopericardium and pneumomediastinum. She had increasing unresponsiveness and died 11 days after admission.

Autopsy examination of the nervous system revealed HIV subacute encephalitis concurrent with cytomegalovirus encephalomyelitis. Microglial nodules, associated with multinucleated giant cells, were evi-

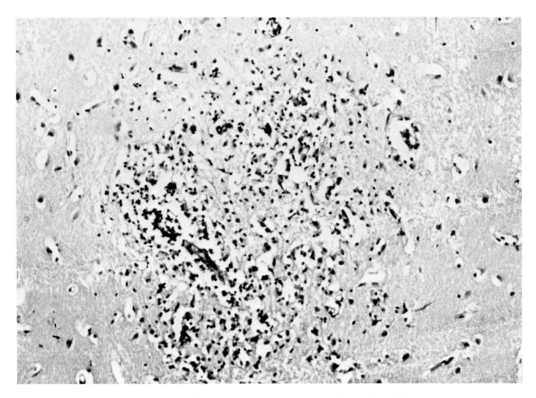

Fig. 6-2. Large microglial nodule in the basal ganglia of a child with AIDS encephalopathy. Microglial nuclei are darkly staining. (Hematoxylin and eosin stain, original magnification ×160.)

dent in the cerebral cortex, cerebral white matter, basal ganglia, brain stem, and cerebellum. The brain exhibited decreased white matter volume and hydrocephalus. Perivascular mineralization was evident in the putamen and, to a lesser extent, in the cerebral white matter (Plate 6-3).

CMV encephalitis was associated with extensive ependymal denudation, subependymal necrosis, and cytomegalic cells with intranuclear and intracytoplasmic inclusions about the ventricles. Subpial necrosis was also prominent in the midbrain, medulla oblongata, and cervical spinal cord. Microglial nodules with cytomegalic cells were evident even in the spinal cord about the central canal.

This infant exhibited the typical course and pathologic findings of congenital HIV infection. The signs of HIV encephalopathy evident in this patient included microglial nodules and multinucleated giant cells. Perivascular calcifications were also evident (Plate 6-4). More than one destructive process can proceed in the central nervous system of AIDS victims, as evidenced by this child's fulminant CMV ependymitis and encephalitis coexisting with an HIV subacute encephalitis. Death in this child was probably from sepsis, despite the extensive central nervous system disease.

Cerebrospinal fluid cultures are often unrevealing in children with early-onset or congenital AIDS.[7] This suggests, but does not prove, that the most common cause of progressive encephalopathy in infants and children with AIDS is HIV, rather than opportunistic infections. As discussed in Chapter 3, the HIV coat protein, gp120, may have toxicity of its own and interfere with the growth and development of neurons.[32] Because neuronal growth is still going on at a rapid pace in newborns and infants, the effect of HIV and its component parts on neurons, if any, would be different from those evident in older children and adults in whom less neuronal development is occurring.[32] That neurons in patients respond to gp120 with the same kind of developmental retardation that is evident in neurons in culture remains to be established.[33]

SOCIOLOGIC ASPECTS

If a child develops AIDS, the source of the infection must be ascertained. If the child is an infant, the mother should be evaluated for HIV infection even if she is not symptomatic for AIDS. The importance of this testing is to predict the outcome of future pregnancies and to anticipate complications in the infected woman. Although no treatment is currently available that will stop the transmission of AIDS transplacentally, some of the antiviral drugs under development appear capable of interfering with transplacental transmission. If the mother is not infected, then another source of infection must be identified. Most commonly this will prove to be tainted blood or blood products. Occasionally the child will be infected through sexual abuse, a problem more likely in older children than in infants.

Current state policies in the United States bar segregation of infected children from the general population. This has met with considerable popular resistance but is based on the lack of proof that AIDS can be transmitted to other children or adults through routine encounters. If an infected child bit another child or left contaminated materials in school during a nosebleed, the disease might be spread, but no incidents of that sort have occurred. Government policies will undoubtedly evolve as the true communicability of AIDS becomes more evident.

REFERENCES

1. CDC: Revision of the CDC surveillance case definition for acquired immunodeficiency syndrome. MMWR 36:3s, 1987
2. Sharer LR, Epstein LG, Cho E-S, et al: Pathologic features of AIDS encephalopathy in children: evidence for LAV/HTLV-III infection of the brain. Hum Pathol 17:271, 1986
3. Sharer LR, Kapila R: Neuropathologic observations in the acquired immunodeficiency syndrome. Acta Neuropathol 66:188, 1985
4. Epstein LG, Sharer LR, Oleske JM, et al: Neurologic manifestations of human immunodeficiency virus infection in children. Pediatrics 78:678, 1986
5. Epstein LG, Goudsmit J, Paul DA, et al: Expression of human immunodeficiency virus in cerebrospinal fluid of children with progressive encephalopathy. Ann Neurol 21:397, 1987
6. Epstein LG, Sharer LR, Joshi VV, et al: Progressive encephalopathy in children with acquired immune deficiency syndrome. Ann Neurol 17:488, 1985
7. Belman AL, Ultmann MH, Horoupian D, et al: Neurological complications in infants and children with acquired immune deficiency syndrome. Ann Neurol 18:560, 1985
8. Jovaisas E, Koch MA, Schafer A, et al: LAV/HTLV-III in 20-week fetus. Lancet 2:129, 1985
9. Lapointe N, Michaud J, Pekovic D, et al: Transplacental transmission of HTLV-III virus. N Engl J Med 312:1325, 1985
10. Marx JL: Spread of AIDS sparks new health concern. Science 219:42, 1983
11. Cowan MJ, Hellmann D, Chudwin D, et al: Maternal transmission of acquired immune deficiency syndrome. Pediatrics 73:382, 1984
12. Gilmer E, Fischer A, Griscelli C, et al: Possible transmission of human lymphotropic retrovirus (LAV) from mother to infant with AIDS. Lancet 1:229, 1984

13. Joncas JH, Delage G, Chad Z, et al: Acquired (or congenital) immunodeficiency syndrome in infants born of Haitian mothers. N Engl J Med 308:842, 1983
14. Hilgartner MW: AIDS and hemophilia. N Engl J Med 317:1153, 1987
15. Wykoff RF, Pearl ER, Saulsbury FT: Immunologic dysfunction in infants infected through transfusion with HTLV-III. N Engl J Med 312:294, 1985
16. Rogers MF: AIDS in children: a review of the clinical, epidemiologic and public health aspects. Pediatr Infect Dis 4:230, 1985
17. Ziegler JB, Cooper DA, Johnson RO, et al: Postnatal transmission of AIDS-associated retrovirus from mother to infant. Lancet 1:896, 1985
18. Pyun KH, Ochs HD, Dufford MTW, Wedgwood RJ: Perinatal infection with human immunodeficiency virus: specific antibody responses by the neonate. N Engl J Med 317:611, 1987
19. Scott GB, Fischl MA, Klimas N, et al: Mothers of infants with acquired immunodeficiency syndrome: evidence for both symptomatic and asymptomatic carriers. JAMA 253:363, 1985
20. Luzi G, Ensoli B, Turbessi G, et al: Transmission of HTLV-III infection by heterosexual contact. Lancet 2:1018, 1985
21. Allain J-P, Laurian Y, Paul DA, et al: Long-term evaluation of HIV antigen and antibodies to p24 and gp41 in patients with hemophilia. N Engl J Med 317:1114, 1987
22. FDA: Special AIDS issue. FDA Drug Bull 17:14, 1987
23. Gilman S, Bloedel J, Lechtenberg R: Disorders of the Cerebellum. F.A. Davis, Philadelphia, 1981
24. Shannon KM, Ammann AJ: Acquired immune deficiency syndrome in childhood. J Pediatr 106:332, 1985
25. Bale JF: Human cytomegalovirus infection and disorders of the nervous system. Arch Neurol 41:310, 1984
26. Pahwa S, Kaplan M, Fikrig S, et al: Spectrum of human T-cell lymphotropic virus type III infection in children: recognition of symptomatic, asymptomatic, and seronegative patients. JAMA 255:2299, 1986
27. Oleske J, Minnefor A, Cooper R, et al: Immune deficiency syndrome in children. JAMA 249:2345, 1983
28. Scott GB, Buck BE, Leterman JG, et al: Acquired immunodeficiency syndrome in infants. N Engl J Med 310:76, 1984
29. Case 9-1986: A 40-month-old girl with the acquired immunodeficiency syndrome and spinal-cord compression. N Engl J Med 314:629, 1986
30. Brun-Vezinet F, Rouzioux C, Montagnier L, et al: Prevalence of antibodies to lymphadenopathy-associated retrovirus in African patients with AIDS. Science 226:453, 1984
31. Sharer LR, Epstein LG, Cho E-S, Petito CK: HTLV-III and vacuolar myelopathy. N Engl J Med 315:62, 1986
32. Lee MR, Ho DR, Gurney ME: Functional interaction and partial homology between human immunodeficiency virus and neuroleukin. Science 237:1047, 1987
33. Barnes DM: Solo actions of AIDS virus coat. Science 237:971, 1987

7

Treatment and Prevention

Survival after the appearance of central nervous system complications of AIDS has been relatively poor despite aggressive treatment. Patients with a mean survival of 9 months from the first signs of AIDS have a mean survival of only 4.4 months from the first appearance of neurologic signs.[1] The patients do not necessarily die as a direct result of the central nervous system lesions, but the appearance of neurologic signs has grave prognostic implications.[1–3] Death may result from *Pneumocystis carinii* pneumonia, disseminated Kaposi's sarcoma, or sepsis.[1,4] Lethal complications develop as an immediate or remote effect of immune system damage, and so any effective treatment must necessarily interfere with the HIV compromise of the immune system.

With a vaccine or antiviral agent that successfully protects the immune system from HIV, patient survival should increase. What remains uncertain is how effective measures that protect the immune system will be in protecting the nervous system from progressive HIV attack. The antiviral agents currently available, such as zidovudine (AZT, Retrovir) and dideoxycytidine, interfere with the replication of the virus, but relatively little viral replication may be needed to produce slowly progressive neurologic deficits. Truly effective treatment of HIV infection must interfere with the progression of both immune and neurologic disease.

INVESTIGATION OF AIDS PATIENTS

The first step in managing neurologic complications of AIDS is the identification of all the problems. Every patient with HIV infection is at risk for neurologic problems, so no AIDS patients can be dismissed as not susceptible to central or peripheral nervous system disease. The systematic investigation of the patient must start with a thorough history and physical examination (Fig. 7-1). If there is any evidence of dementia, seizure activity, weakness, incoordination, or sensory disturbance, the basis for that finding must be determined quickly. A rapid and thorough investigation may improve the long-term outcome.

Hematologic studies are of less value in the AIDS patient than in other patients with neurologic disturbances because the hematologic picture is usually disturbed by the HIV infection. A raging meningitis need not be associated with an elevated peripheral white blood cell count or even a shift of the differential to more immature forms. If the patient has any evidence of neurologic signs or symptoms, an MRI or CT should be obtained to ascertain if there is a focal structural lesion, such as an abscess or granuloma. If a mass is evident, it should be biopsied.

Patients with evidence of hydrocephalus may require shunting. Ventriculoperitoneal

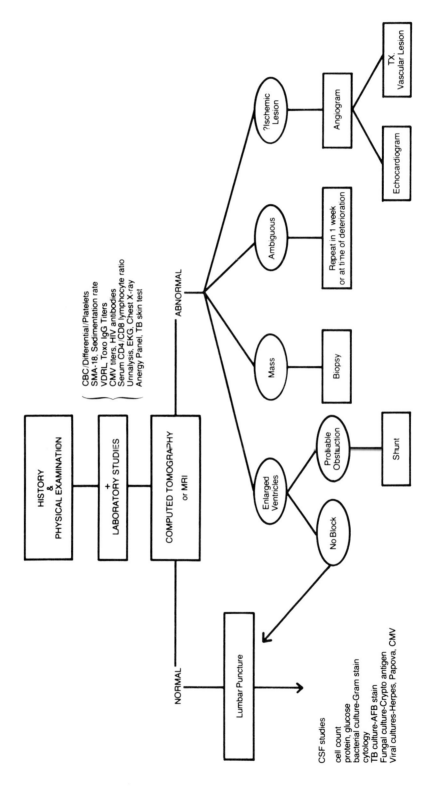

Fig. 7-1. Flow diagram for the investigation of the AIDS patient.

shunt placement should not be delayed if it appears to be required. When the shunt is placed, the surgeon can collect cerebrospinal fluid for further analysis and may obtain a cerebral biopsy to look for HIV subacute encephalitis or early cerebral toxoplasmosis.

Patients with no structural abnormalities on neuroimaging studies should have cerebrospinal fluid analyses to look for infection or tumor. Meningeal lymphomatosis is less likely with primary brain lymphomas than with metastatic lymphomas, but cytologic studies may reveal tumor cells nonetheless. Immunologic studies of the cerebrospinal fluid are now readily available and can be used to check for cryptococcal infection. Any depression of the cerebrospinal fluid glucose should be dealt with as meningitis until there is convincing evidence to the contrary.

If the patient has evidence of intracranial infarction or hemorrhage, more attention must be paid to hematologic parameters and the cardiovascular status of the patient. Valvular heart disease should be specifically sought in the patient who has had infarction. Thrombocytopenia must be looked for in the patient with hemorrhagic lesions, but the possibility of hemorrhage into a tumor must also be considered.

Peripheral nerve studies and electromyography are indicated if there is evidence of denervation or myopathy because AIDS patients are not exempt from routine causes of nerve and muscle disease, such as entrapment syndromes and parasitic infections. Thorough investigation of such possibilities may require sural nerve or skeletal muscle biopsies.

Patients with AIDS have persistent vulnerability to opportunistic infections and tumors, and so repeated evaluations may be necessary. That a patient has no mass from a toxoplasma granuloma 1 week does not guarantee that none will be evident the next month or even the next week. As long as the patient has a deteriorating course, investigations must be repeated frequently until the basis for the deterioration is evident.

One of the dilemmas to be faced as patient survival increases is the evaluation of cerebral masses in previously investigated patients. The morbidity associated with repeated brain biopsies is substantial in immunocompetent patients, but in immunodeficient patients it would be unacceptable. If a nocardial abscess is successfully treated and another brain mass appears, reoperation on the patient carries too low a probability of benefit to justify the procedure. What are needed to avoid repeated explorations of the brain are tests that more specifically identify the character of the intracranial lesion. Magnetic resonance imaging or radionuclide scans may be helpful in differentiating between the different types of intracranial masses, but they are not yet capable of this.

MANAGEMENT OF SYSTEMIC DISEASE

Most patients with neurologic problems and AIDS die from systemic, not neurologic, diseases. Overwhelming sepsis or intractable pneumonia account for most of the deaths in patients with neurologic disease, and so attention must never be diverted by the neurologic problem from the patient's systemic problems.

One of the most obvious systemic effects of AIDS is leukopenia. With the recent availability of blood precursor colony stimulating factors, trials have begun to determine the value of leukocyte inducing agents in individuals with AIDS.[5] Experience with granulocyte-macrophage colony-stimulating factor in these patients has been encouraging. Severely leukopenic patients have had significant increases in their white blood cell counts while they received this colony-stimulating factor.[5]

Some of the complications of AIDS, such

as the thrombocytopenia that often develops, have immunologic bases. Consequently, inappropriate immune activity must be managed in these patients with inadequate immune function. Obviously, successful strategies for managing such systemic problems have not yet been developed and will probably require drugs that irreversibly inhibit the AIDS virus.

TREATMENT OF NEUROLOGIC COMPLICATIONS

Aside from HIV subacute encephalitis, most of the neurologic problems that develop with AIDS are treatable (Table 7-1). However, what can be effectively treated in patients without AIDS need not respond to treatment in patients with AIDS. The immune deficiency state limits the effectiveness of antibiotic regimens and increases

Table 7-1. Treatment of Central Nervous System Complications of AIDS

Disorder	Treatment
HIV subacute encephalomyelitis	Zidovudine
HIV or idiopathic meningitis	Zidovudine
Herpes simplex encephalitis	Acyclovir or adenine arabinoside
Cytomegalovirus	Vidarabine and interferon
Progressive multifocal leucoencephalopathy	Cytarabine
Toxoplasma gondii	Pyramethamine + Sulfadiazine
Cryptococcus neoformans	Amphotericin B + 5-Flucytosine
Candida albicans	Amphotericin B
Coccidioidomycosis	Amphotericin B
Syphilis	Penicillin
Atypical mycobacteria	INH, ethambutol, rifampin, clofazimine
Mycobacterium tuberculosis	INH, ethambutol, rifampin
Nocardia asteroides	Trimethoprim + sulfamethoxazole
Primary CNS lymphoma	Neuraxis radiation
Metastatic CNS lymphoma	Radiation, chemotherapy
Kaposi's sarcoma	Radiation, chemotherapy
Embolic stroke	Treat etiology
Hemorrhagic stroke	Treat etiology

the probability of recurrent lesions. Until a treatment becomes available that thoroughly reverses the damage done by the retrovirus, measures to restrain the effects of opportunistic infections and AIDS-associated brain tumors can never be more than partially effective.

The attack on the brain itself by HIV requires that any agent developed for the treatment of AIDS be able to work in the brain. This means that antiviral agents developed must be able to cross the blood-brain barrier and not produce neurotoxicity.[6] Because children may carry HIV in the brain for months or years before progressive disease begins, agents developed to eliminate the neurologic damage done by the AIDS virus will need to be given before the patient is symptomatic.[6] Lifelong therapy probably will be needed to deal with the latent virus or provirus residing in the central nervous system.[6]

ANTIVIRAL AGENTS

Several agents believed to interfere with viral replication have been tested for their effectiveness against HIV. One of the major constraints on the antiviral therapies is that the drugs used must be able to cross the blood-brain barrier and reach effective concentrations in the central nervous system.[7] Antiviral agents available before the AIDS epidemic started that could enter the brain included zidovudine (AZT) and ribavirin.[7] The only drug to consistently improve the outcome in patients with AIDS has been zidovudine (AZT), but because it does not eliminate all morbidity and mortality in patients with AIDS and does not interfere with acquisition of the disease, a variety of other drugs and vaccines are being developed.

Zidovudine (AZT)

Zidovudine (azidothymidine, AZT, Retrovir) is effective in the treatment of patients with AIDS, even after they have developed signs of neurologic disease.[8,9] This drug unequivocally reduces the death rate and incidence of opportunistic infections in patients with AIDS, but it does not halt the disease or prevent its spread to uninfected individuals. It is a thymidine analogue, its chemical structure being 3'-azido-3'-deoxy-thymidine (Fig. 7-2).[8,10] As a thymidine analogue it inhibits the reverse transcriptase that is essential for the AIDS virus to successfully infect cells.[8] The triphosphate of zidovudine is substituted for thymidine in the process that converts the viral RNA to DNA, thereby interrupting the elongation of the proviral DNA chain.[8,10]

Aside from reducing the patient death rate, this drug increases the number of CD4 T lymphocytes surviving in treated individuals.[8] Recovery of delayed hypersensitivity reactions and weight gain have also been observed in patients treated with this drug, both of which are objective signs of immune system recovery.[9]

Zidovudine has been approved for use in AIDS victims who have had *Pneumocystis carinii* pneumonia or have a CD4 T lymphocyte count of less than 200 cells per μL.[11] It requires doses four times a day for months at a time and produces anemia in many of the patients to whom it is administered.[12] The recommended starting dose is 200 mg every 4 hours. This dose may need to be adjusted if severe toxicity develops.

The first significant decrease in the rate of opportunistic infections observed in treated patients does not develop until after 6 weeks of treatment.[8] Virus can still be cultured from patients after several months of zidovudine treatment, so they must be considered at risk of transmitting the disease.[8] This drug has no demonstrable efficacy against the other viruses that may infect the AIDS patient opportunistically, such as papovaviruses and herpesviruses. If infection with these viruses is reduced, it is because cellular immunity recovers.

Toxic effects of zidovudine include bone marrow suppression with macrocytosis, anemia, and neutropenia.[12,13] Patients complain of nausea, myalgia, insomnia, and headache but are rarely so intolerant of the drug as to require cessation of treatment.[12] Hematologic complications occur most often in patients who start treatment after severe hematologic problems are already evident.[12] A low-serum vitamin B_{12} level at

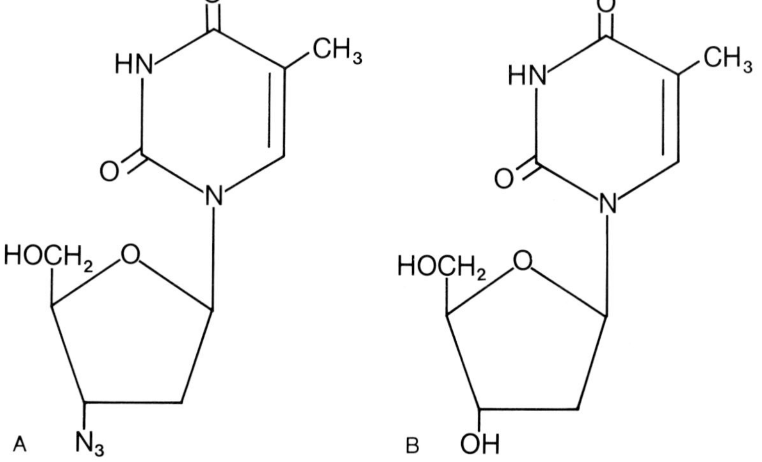

Fig. 7-2. Chemical structure of zidovudine (**A**) compared to thymidine (**B**). The only difference between the compounds is the substitution of an azido group for the hydroxyl group on thymidine.

the start of therapy correlates with a high incidence of neutropenia as a complication of treatment.[12] There is reason to wonder about the carcinogenic or mutagenic effects of this drug, but a clear demonstration of its safety has been bypassed in efforts to distribute a drug effective against AIDS.[13]

Zidovudine crosses the blood-brain barrier well. Its level in the cerebrospinal fluid of patients with active infection is about half of that in the serum. It has no deleterious effect on cognitive or affective function. Patients with minor cognitive deficits have shown slightly improved performance on memory tasks.[14] Affective flattening is not substantially reversed.

That any improvement at all in cognitive function is seen in patients treated with zidovudine supports the notion that HIV does not kill neurons.[15] Studies with cell cultures have raised questions about the toxicity to neurons of the retrovirus or of its component parts.[16] That improvement occurs with zidovudine treatment indicates that all of the cognitive dysfunction observed in AIDS patients does not occur as a result of neuronal damage, but it does not eliminate the possibility that neuronal damage, rather than just neuronal dysfunction, does occur.

At least in experimental animals, zidovudine crosses the placenta and interferes with the progression of retroviral injury to the fetus,[17] but this has yet to be confirmed in pregnant women. Toxic effects on non-human fetuses appear to be negligible.

Dideoxycytidine (DDC)

2′,3′-dideoxycytidine (DDC) acts in a manner similar to zidovudine in inhibiting the action of reverse transcriptase as it creates the DNA provirus, but precisely what it does in infected cells and can do in uninfected cells is unknown.[13] Toxicity studies have yet to be completed.

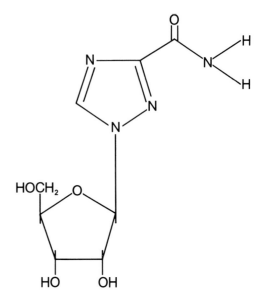

Fig. 7-3. Ribavirin.

Ribavirin

Ribavirin is a purine nucleoside analogue capable of inhibiting some RNA viruses[18] (Fig. 7-3). Ribavirin inhibits replication of HIV in vitro, but when used in combination with zidovudine, it antagonizes the effectiveness of zidovudine.[10] It appears that this antiviral agent may delay or prevent the development of AIDS in patients with persistent lymphadenopathy secondary to HIV.[10] It has been used in combination with interferon-alpha A and appears to inhibit synergistically in vitro HIV replication.[10]

Ribavirin remains active and available when it is taken orally and does cross the blood-brain barrier.[10] It is phosphorylated intracellularly, and the triphosphate of ribavirin interferes with posttranscriptional processing.[19] In clinical trials, it has significantly delayed the progression of HIV-associated lymphadenopathy to AIDS.[10]

Peptide T

In Sweden and the United States, limited trials have been conducted using a protein presumed to interfere with the entry of

D-Ala-Ser-Thr-Thr-Thr-Asn-Tyr-Thr-NH$_2$

Fig. 7-4. Peptide T.

HIV-1 into the cell. This is called protein T or peptide T and is a short segment of the glycoprotein gp120 normally occurring in the HIV envelope[20,21] (Fig. 7-4). Peptide T is derived from gp120, the envelope glycoprotein of HIV-1.[22] Some researchers believe that it interferes with the binding of the virus to the docking site, the T4 or CD4 antigen, on cells that become infected.[20–22] Whether it has any effect on viral binding, spread, or replication is still debatable.[22]

The original rationale for using the peptide was that it represented an element in the virus envelope that was highly conserved from strain to strain, but this view has been discredited by studies on highly variable virus coats.[22] Recent studies on the binding of the viral coat to the receptor antigen indicate that three separate segments of the glycoprotein gp120 are needed for binding and none of those three include the peptide T segment.[20] This does not mean that peptide T is necessarily ineffective at inhibiting the binding, but it does undermine the rationale for its use in clinical trials. Few patients have been treated, but the protein does appear to improve survival without causing additional complications. Studies done to date have involved few patients and have been uncontrolled.[22]

Other Approaches

Combinations of various antiviral regimens are being tested. Tumor necrosis factor and gamma interferon are being used in one trial. Gamma interferon strongly inhibits virus expression from latently infected promonocyte cells.[23] Whether this or any of the other agent currently being tested will be of substantial value in reducing morbidity and mortality from AIDS remains to be

seen. The most promising, but most complex, antiviral approaches involve manipulation of the genetic code or regulator genes in the AIDS virus itself. If the genetic composition of the virus can be used against itself, either by destroying vital elements of the genome or activating genes at inappropriate times, the virus may be defeated. As the regulatory and structural genes that constitute the virus are better understood, the feasibility of such approaches increases.

Antineoplastic Measures

Neoplasms that develop with AIDS will not necessarily remit when HIV is effectively managed. It is possible, but unlikely, that the primary brain lymphomas and metastatic Kaposi's sarcoma seen in these patients will occur even after the immune system damage caused by the retrovirus is controlled. If they do persist, they will require measures aimed specifically at them. These would include radiation therapy to the entire craniospinal axis and chemotherapy.

COUNSELING

When patients are told that they have AIDS, they usually respond with denial or disbelief. This yields within days or weeks to depression and anxiety.[24] Many patients complain of hopelessness and fearful uncertainty, and some become suicidal. As part of the anxiety that attends the diagnosis, patients complain of agitation, loss of appetite, insomnia, and palpitations.[24] Also very much a part of the response to the diagnosis is anger directed toward a variety of targets, including governments that are not vigorously dealing with the disease, individuals who disparage high risk groups, and medical institutions who provide no cure for the disease.[24] In many ways, the patient's reaction to the diagnosis is typical of the reaction to any diagnosis that confers upon the individual an untreatable, terminal disease.

Designating an individual as having AIDS-related complex, rather than AIDS, does little to lessen the impact of the verdict. Most individuals who are told they have AIDS-related complex soon learn that they are at substantial risk of developing AIDS and respond with the same anger and depression exhibited by the patient with AIDS.

Complicating the psychiatric problems experienced by patients with AIDS is the social isolation that is likely to ensue once the diagnosis becomes known. This isolation may exacerbate the guilt associated with having developed this disease, a guilt experienced by many patients developing a life threatening disease.[24] With AIDS the feeling of guilt is linked to activities, such as drug use or homosexual activity, that placed the individual at increased risk, but what the guilt is associated with is less important in management than that the patient is burdened by guilt. The combination of this guilt with depression or dementia increases the risk of self-destructive behavior. Frankly self-destructive acts including suicide are occurring with disturbing frequency, especially in men who survive several months with AIDS.[24]

Programs for counseling AIDS victims and their families are an essential component of any treatment plan. Discussion groups are often helpful in defusing stressful issues and in developing strategies for coping with the disease as well as possible. Antidepressants are appropriate if the patient develops a reactive depression, but any significant depression should be considered to be a sign of neurologic disease unless it is established to be otherwise.

The management of AIDS is also complicated by the reaction of medical staff to the disease.[25] The fear of acquiring the disease is as substantial for health care workers as it is for the general public. Working in close contact with victims of AIDS is distressing for these workers, not only because they worry about acquiring the virus, but also because the patients they are caring for may be from social groups, such as homosexuals and intravenous drug abusers, against which they harbor strong prejudices. Also contributing to stress in the interactions between health care workers and the patients is the perception that these are terminally ill individuals. All of these problems should be anticipated and discussed frankly with the workers coming into contact with the patients. Strategies for minimizing the stress faced by the workers will improve the care ultimately received by the patients.

PREVENTION

The neurologic consequences of HIV infection and of AIDS can be avoided with certainty only if the virus is eliminated from all currently infected populations. This obviously can be done, as was demonstrated with smallpox, if an effective vaccine is widely available and containment of the infectious agent is vigorously enforced. With HIV neither condition has been fulfilled. There is no effective vaccine, and there is no organized effort being made to sequester the infectious agent.[11] Now that the disease is an international problem, a coordinated international effort will be needed to eliminate it. Based on experience with other infectious agents, many options are available that would reliably affect the spread of the virus, but most have proved politically unacceptable. Because of the failure of epidemiologic options, considerable effort is being directed toward the development of a vaccine.

The simplest strategy in any epidemic caused by personal or tissue contact is to sequester the affected individuals and screen rigorously for infected materials, such as blood or organs. Programs to identify HIV carriers have met with resistance, so personal contact cannot be avoided. Because the principal routes of infection have been through sexual contact and sharing of needles for intravenous injection, several programs have been fostered in the United States to dissuade all members of the population from engaging in a variety of sexual practices thought to increase the risk of acquiring the virus and to dissuade drug addicts from sharing needles. Both campaigns are affecting the behavior of the targeted populations, but neither is substantially slowing the spread of infection within those populations.

Blood Testing

Testing of blood and blood products has become routine.[11] The ELISA test used to detect antibodies to HIV is relatively inexpensive, simple to perform, and widely available. Using this test to check blood and blood products will reduce the rate of spread of the virus through transfusion but will not have a major impact on the spread of AIDS because transfusions have contributed only slightly to the spread of the disease. It will reduce the risk to patients requiring frequent infusions of blood and blood products, such as hemophiliacs. Unfortunately, most of the hemophiliacs receiving pooled blood products between 1980 and 1985 were exposed to the virus. For newly diagnosed hemophiliacs, the probability of receiving tainted blood products is considerably less than for the group exposed before 1985, but there is still a small risk that antibody negative samples will have viable HIV.[11]

The risk of acquiring AIDS through transfusion is now exceedingly small, perhaps less than 1 in 100,000; but that there is any risk is a strong inducement for using autologous blood whenever feasible. Autologous blood is collected from the patient and

transfused back in when needed. This is usually practical in cases of elective surgery, but much of the blood supply in the United States and Europe is used for emergency surgery.

Quarantine

With reassurances from medical experts, the courts in the United States have consistently ruled against isolating individuals with AIDS, whether it be in school or in the workplace. This policy will almost certainly prove justified over the next decade, but it is based on projections from the data available, rather than on protracted experience with the disease.[11] In New York City and many other cities in the United States where the issue has been argued in court, children with AIDS are placed in public schools without being identified, so students, teachers, and school health officials have no way of knowing with which children they must use precautions. In case of a bloody nose or a cut lip, every child must be dealt with as a possible HIV carrier. This imposes burdens on the school systems that are simply being ignored.

Contact Precautions

Health care workers are becoming more sophisticated in their handling of patients with AIDS.[11] Protective gloves, gowns, and masks are finding increasing acceptance among laboratory, nursing, and housekeeping staff members.[25-27] Physicians operating on AIDS patients are also using protective eye gear, such as goggles, on a regular basis. Barriers to routine screening of patients admitted to hospitals still complicate the handling of blood and tissue specimens obtained during hospitalization.

Sexual Precautions

The most common route for transmission of the virus is through sexual contact, so this must be a prime focus for any policies aimed at reducing dissemination of the virus. Several measures do appear to reduce sexual transmission of the virus. Latex condoms interfere with the introduction of sperm into the vagina or rectum and limit the exposure of the urethra to vaginal secretions or rectal contents during intercourse.[28,29] If current ideas about how the virus is transmitted during sexual activity are accurate, latex condoms should provide an effective barrier both to transmission and acquisition of the virus.[11] Several widely available spermicidal agents, such as nonoxynol-9, inactivate the virus, so use of such spermicidal agents should increase the margin of safety during sexual intercourse. Anal intercourse is associated with a higher risk of viral transmission and should be discouraged in heterosexual relationships. Sexual activity when either partner has a venereal infection, such as syphilis, gonorrhea, or chlamydia, increases the risk of acquisition, and so this too should be avoided.

Unfortunately, legislation in any area relating to sexual education or activity has always faced very stiff public resistance in the United States. The result is that initiatives to promote the use of condoms by men and nonoxynol-9 by both men and women have been consistently thwarted. Discussions of changes in sexual activity have been limited to recommendations that people never have sexual intercourse outside marriage. Policy statements at state and national levels have been remarkably timid and naive.

VACCINATION

With the current understanding of AIDS, the only practical way of stopping the spread of the disease is with a vaccine. Several characteristics of HIV are hindering the development of such a vaccine.[11,30] One problem is that this is a retrovirus that affects humans in a very different way from that in which it affects other animals.[31] The genetic material is RNA, not DNA, and it is genetically complex. The HIV can mutate to a great number of variants, perhaps even after it enters the body.[32,33] Any vaccine developed must take into account this variability and must also be able to deal with the virus whether it attacks the body as a free particle or within a cell infected with the virus.[34] HIV can enter the body completely hidden inside infected cells, a trait not previously dealt with in vaccine development.[30] Once in the body it may spread from cell to cell by direct cell contact rather than through intermediate phases as free virions.[30] Vaccines cannot act against a virus that does not expose itself outside the infected cell.

Ordinarily, antibodies formed against a virus would bind to specific viral proteins and trigger further immune reactions. Vaccines prepare the immune system to respond rapidly to viral antigens by exposing them to harmless forms of the antigen. Vaccines have traditionally been made from inactivated virus or innocuous strains of virus. Ways to reliably and irreversibly inactivate HIV while preserving its ability to elicit an effective antigenic response are not currently available. It is also not clear that there are any truly harmless variants of HIV. Further complicating vaccine development is the presence of oncogene promoter segments in HIV. This means than some of the nucleic acids that the virus has can lead to cancerous tumors if they produce DNA that inserts near oncogenes.

Current efforts are focusing on isolating specific genes from HIV that code for proteins that might prove strategic if infection occurs. The proteins that are produced in quantity from transplants of these genes to other organisms would be tried as part of the vaccine. An alternative approach involves splicing a harmless HIV gene into vaccinia virus. Vaccinia is familiar to healthcare workers all over the world, and it is a relatively large virus. Its size allows the insertion of many genes, if that should prove necessary.

What remains unknown is what will constitute an effective vaccine. People infected with HIV have developed neutralizing antibodies but still have developed AIDS.[30] Even with antibodies against the virus, infection can get into the body in infected cells and can travel into highly sequestered regions, such as the central nervous system, regions that antibodies may have difficulty reaching. If the vaccine only serves to interfere with the transmissibility of the virus it still will be useful for the general population, even if it provides little protection to each individual.[32]

Several conventional and unconventional studies are currently under way in an effort to develop a vaccine against HIV infection. One physician inoculated himself and volunteers from Zaire with recombinant vaccinia virus containing a gene from the AIDS virus.[35] The rationale for the vaccination was to use the AIDS gene to trigger signals that would promote cell mediated immunity against different subtypes of the AIDS virus.[35] The gene used in this vaccine is the one coding for the envelope glycoprotein. The initial immune response did produce antibodies against the viral subtype from which the gene was taken, but these antibodies did not neutralize other isolates.[35] However, the vaccine did stimulate lymphocyte mitosis and expression of T-cell receptors for interleukin 2 when the lymphocytes from vaccinated individuals were exposed to different viral isolates in vitro.[35] Both of these are cell mediated responses.[35] This same physician also attempted to treat already infected patients by injecting them with formaldehyde-fixed cells that had previously been infected with the virus. His rationale was to present antigen from the virus in a form that was not infectious.[35]

Other strategies for developing a vaccine have focused on the precursor of the viral envelope protein, gp160.[36,37] This glycoprotein includes the gp120 component of the outer viral coat and the gp41 component that spans the viral envelope membrane. This glycoprotein precursor can be inserted into vaccinia viruses and thereby used to elicit an antibody response to the HIV coat protein. One vaccine already being used in trials uses a modified viral coat gene that has been inserted into baculovirus, a virus that infects moths and butterflies.[37] This engineered virus can be grown in insect cells. A variety of animals innoculated with this virus produce antibodies that block HIV replication in cultured human T lymphocytes.[37] This experimental vaccine also stimulates cell-mediated immunity.

Chimpanzees are the only primates that can be infected with HIV, although they do not develop AIDS as it appears in humans.[36] Experience with vaccination of these animals has been worrisome because they do mount immune responses to HIV and yet still have evidence of intracellular infection.[36,37]

An alternative approach is to use anti-idiotypes, antibodies to antibodies. An antigen is injected into an animal, the animal develops antibodies to the antigen, and then these antibodies are injected into another animal and antibodies to the antibodies are produced. This technique could be used to produce antibodies to the receptor sites, but this may present new problems, since the CD4 receptor is found in many different tissues including the central nervous system.

The 9,264 nucleotide sequence of the HIV-like virus that is found in African green monkeys has been completely determined and is very similar to HIV-2, the virus commonly causing AIDS in West Africa.[31] This simian virus is more remotely related to HIV-1, the cause of AIDS in the United States.[31] The African green monkey virus is called STLV-III. Comparisons of these three different viruses have been helpful in identifying the constant features of the genetic material that account for the various properties of the viruses in different animals. Some of the regions on the virus genome are remarkably highly conserved, although these retroviruses typically vary considerably from strain to strain. These constant elements are presumed to underlie the infectivity of the virus.[31] The constant nucleotide sequences in the genome may code for an essential element in the attack mechanism of the virus and may provide ideal sites for blocking viral action.[31]

Also vital to the development of a vaccine is the discovery of an HIV-like retrovirus (SIV-1) that actually causes an AIDS-like disease in macaque monkeys.[31] This is a different strain of STLV-III from that which affects African green monkeys and is more different from HIV than the green monkey STLV-III, but its induction of immunodeficiency in a primate allows for controlled experiments that until now have been impractical.

Along less conventional lines, some investigators have used yeast DNA with the ability to produce virus-like particles to create packets of protein that include multiple copies of HIV antigen.[38] The special DNA accepts segments of DNA typical of the AIDS provirus.[38] It then produces packets of protein with various noninfectious components of HIV. These virus-like particles with genetic material can be used as a vaccine.

PROGNOSIS

AIDS is not the first devastating viral illness, and it is not even the first lethal viral illness that causes neurologic problems.[18] When the measles virus came out of Africa with one of the many military campaigns waged against southern Europe by Islamic forces during the Middle Ages, tens of millions of people died from neurologic complications of the viral illness. Other epidemics have spread across continents, more often spread by trade than by war, with loss of life that dwarfs the AIDS epidemic. However, the disconcerting aspect of AIDS is not the novelty of this type of infection, but rather the ineffectiveness of modern countermeasures.

Viral epidemics have been increasingly viewed as manageable. Intractable spread of such a lethal disease was generally dismissed as a problem resolved decades ago. Poliomyelitis was the last great challenge, and modern medicine triumphed. Few outside of virology appreciate how limited is the arsenal for dealing with lethal epidemics and how likely the appearance of new viral killers continues to be.

The AIDS epidemic will end simply because all such epidemics end. How many people will die or suffer devastating neurologic injury before this virus follows the route followed by all such lethal infections is unknowable. The most important determinant of the toll that this virus will take is the speed with which countermeasures are developed. Without any medical intervention, the epidemic will run its course and disappear, perhaps in 5 years, perhaps in 50 years. This has always been true with highly lethal viral illnesses; indeed, this has always been true with retroviruses.

The epidemic is not raging onward as indiscriminately as it appeared inclined to be doing when it was first recognized. In the American cities most dramatically affected, such as New York and San Francisco, the epidemic is not spreading substantially beyond those high risk groups identified early in the epidemic.[39] Heterosexual women and strictly heterosexual men are rarely developing AIDS unless they are abusing drugs or receiving tainted blood products.

What is disturbing is that progressive neurologic damage has proven to be a major component of the disease. This neurologic component may also prove to be the most refractory to treatment. Even if strategies are developed that minimize the immune system damage inflicted by the virus, progressive neurologic deterioration may still appear in HIV infected individuals. That an effective vaccine can be developed with the technology currently available to virologists is less certain now than in 1983 when AIDS was accepted as a syndrome caused by a virus. That neurologic disease will be stopped by anything less than a vaccine that prevents infection with the virus is unlikely. AIDS, the human immunodeficiency virus, and its effects on the nervous system will pose continuing dilemmas for physicians at least over the next decade.

REFERENCES

1. Levy RM, Pons VG, Rosenblum ML: Intracerebral mass lesions in the acquired immunodeficiency syndrome (AIDS). J Neurosurg 61:9, 1984
2. Koppel BS, Wormser GP, Tuchman AJ, et al: Central nervous system involvement in patients with acquired immunodeficiency syndrome. Acta Neurol Scand 71:337, 1985
3. Welch K, Finkbeiner W, Alpers CE, et al: Autopsy findings in the acquired immune deficiency syndrome. JAMA 252:1152, 1984
4. Anders KH, Guerra WF, Tomiyasu U, et al: The neuropathology of AIDS. UCLA experience and review. Am J Pathol 124:537, 1986
5. Groopman JE, Mitsuyasu RT, DeLeo MJ, et al: Effect of recombinant human granulocyte-macrophage colony-stimulating factor on myelopoiesis in the acquired immunodeficiency syndrome. N Engl J Med 317:593, 1987
6. Epstein LG, Sharer LR, Oleske JM, et al: Neurologic manifestations of human immunodeficiency virus infection in children. Pediatrics 78:678, 1986
7. Gabuzda DH, Kirsch MS: Neurologic manifestations of infection with human immunodeficiency virus. Ann Intern Med 107:383–391, 1987
8. Fischl MA, Richman DD, Grieco MH, et al: The efficacy of azidothymidine (AZT) in the treatment of patients with AIDS and AIDS-related complex. N Engl J Med 317:185, 1987
9. Yarchoan R, Broder S: Development of antiretroviral therapy for the acquired immunodeficiency syndrome and related disorders: a progress report. N Engl J Med 316:557, 1987
10. Vogt MW, Hartshorn KL, Furman PA, et al: Ribavirin antagonizes the effect of azidothymidine on HIV replication. Science 235:1376, 1987
11. FDA: Special AIDS issue. FDA Drug Bull 17:14, 1987
12. Richman DD, Fischl MA, Grieco MH, et al: The toxicity of azidothymidine (AZT) in the treatment of patients with AIDS and AIDS-related complex. N Engl J Med 317:192, 1987
13. Cohen SS: Antiretroviral therapy for AIDS. N Engl J Med 317:629, 1987
14. Edwards DD: 'Competition' cause of AIDS dementia? Science News 132:150, 1987
15. Barnes DM: Solo actions of AIDS virus coat. Science 237:971, 1987
16. Lee MR, Ho DR, Gurney ME: Functional interaction and partial homology between human immunodeficiency virus and neuroleukin. Science 237:1047, 1987
17. Sharpe AH, Jaenisch R, Ruprecht RM: Retroviruses and mouse embryos: A rapid model for neurovirulence and transplacental antiviral therapy. Science 236:1671, 1987
18. Johnson RT: Viral Infections of The Nervous System. Raven Press, New york, 1982
19. Gilbert BE, Knight V: Antimicrob Agents Chemother 30:201, 1986
20. Marx JL: Probing the AIDS virus and its relatives. Science 236:1523, 1987
21. Pert CB, Hill JM, Ruff MR, et al: Octopeptides deduced from neuropeptide receptor-like pattern of antigen T4 in brain potently inhibit human immunodeficiency virus receptor binding and T-cell infectivity. Proc Natl Acad Sci USA 83:9254, 1986
22. Barnes DM: Debate over potential AIDS drug. Science 237:128, 1987
23. Barnes DM: Cytokines alter AIDS virus production. Science 236:1627, 1987
24. Marzuk PM, Tierney H, Tardiff K, et al: Increased risk of suicide in persons with AIDS. JAMA 259:1333, 1988

25. CDC: Update: human immunodeficiency virus infections in health-care workers exposed to blood of infected patients. MMWR 36:285, 1987

26. CDC: Recommendations for preventing transmission of infection with human T-lymphotropic virus type III/lymphadenopathy-associated virus in the workplace. MMWR 34:682, 691, 1985

27. CDC: Recommended infection-control practices for dentistry. MMWR 35:237, 1986

28. Conant M, et al: Condoms prevent transmission of AIDS-associated retrovirus. JAMA 255:1706, 1986

29. Mann J, Quinn TC, Piot P, et al: Condom use and HIV infection among prostitutes in Zaire. N Engl J Med 316:345, 1987

30. Marx JL: The AIDS virus—well known but a mystery. Science 236:390, 1987

31. Weiss R: AIDS vaccine: research on target. Science News 132:84, 1987

32. Barnes DM: Broad issues debated at AIDS vaccine workshop. Science 236:255, 1987

33. Anand R, Siegal F, Reed C, et al: Non-cytocidal natural variants of human immunodeficiency virus isolated from AIDS patients with neurological disorders. Lancet 2:234, 1987

34. Edwards DD: High-risk sex studied in women, men. Science News 132:116, 1987

35. Barnes DM: Candidate AIDS vaccine. Science 235:1575, 1987

36. Edwards DD: Human test of AIDS vaccine approved. Science News 132:116, 1987

37. Barnes DM: AIDS vaccine trial OKed. Science 237:973, 1987

38. Edwards DD: Hybrid particle mimics AIDS virus. Science News 132:151, 1987

39. Sande M: Transmission of AIDS: the case against contagion. N Engl J Med 341:380, 1986

Index

Page numbers followed by t represent tables; those followed by f represent figures; pl refers to plate numbers rather than page numbers.

138 • Index